F*ck Fibro

A pain tracking journal

WELLNESS WARRIOR PRESS

Copyright © 2020 by Wellness Warrior Press

ISBN: 978-0-9813530-0-5

This journal belongs to...

_____

DOCTOR / SPECIALIST INFORMATION

Name	Address	Contact

DAILY MEDICATION / SUPPLEMENTS

Medication / Supplement	Dosage

Summary

For each journal entry, return to this summary page and
rate your overall pain / discomfort level
(1 being no pain and 10 being unbearable)

Entry #	Rating	Entry #	Rating
1		31	
2		32	
3		33	
4		34	
5		35	
6		36	
7		37	
8		38	
9		39	
10		40	
11		41	
12		42	
13		43	
14		44	
15		45	
16		46	
17		47	
18		48	
19		49	
20		50	
21		51	
22		52	
23		53	
24		54	
25		55	
26		56	
27		57	
28		58	
29		59	
30		60	

Date: _____

How are you feeling today?

Like death	Like shit	Not good	Meh	Good	Great!	Amazing!

RATE YOUR PAIN LEVEL

① ② ③ ④ ⑤ ⑥ ⑦ ⑧ ⑨ ⑩

Describe your pain / symptoms

	am	pm
	☐	☐
	☐	☐
	☐	☐
	☐	☐
	☐	☐
	☐	☐
	☐	☐
	☐	☐

Where do you feel it?

Front   *Back*

What about your...?

Mood	① ② ③ ④ ⑤ ⑥ ⑦ ⑧ ⑨ ⑩
Energy levels	① ② ③ ④ ⑤ ⑥ ⑦ ⑧ ⑨ ⑩
Mental clarity	① ② ③ ④ ⑤ ⑥ ⑦ ⑧ ⑨ ⑩

Feeling sick?

☐ Nope!
☐ Yes...

☐ Nausea   ☐ Diarrhea   ☐ Vomiting   ☐ Sore throat
☐ Congestion   ☐ Coughing   ☐ Chills   ☐ Fever

Other symptoms: _____

| Hours of Sleep | ① ② ③ ④ ⑤ ⑥ ⑦ ⑧ ⑨ ⑩ ⊕ |
| Sleep Quality | ① ② ③ ④ ⑤ ⑥ ⑦ ⑧ ⑨ ⑩ |

WEATHER

☐ Hot   ☐ Mild   ☐ Cold   BM Pressure: _____

☐ Dry   ☐ Humid   ☐ Wet   Allergen Levels: _____

STRESS LEVELS

| None | Low | Medium | High | Max | @$#%! |

FOOD / MEDICATIONS

FOOD / DRINKS	MEDS / SUPPLEMENTS	TIME	DOSE

☐ usual daily medication

EXERCISE / DAILY ACTIVITY

☐ Damn right, I worked out.

☐ I managed to exercise a bit.

☐ No, I haven't exercised at all.

☐ I did some stuff, and that counts.

DETAILS

NOTES / TRIGGERS / IMPROVEMENTS

_____

_____

_____

WRITE ONE THING YOU'RE GRATEFUL FOR

_____

Date: _____

How are you feeling today?

| Like death | Like shit | Not good | Meh | Good | Great! | Amazing! |

RATE YOUR PAIN LEVEL

① ② ③ ④ ⑤ ⑥ ⑦ ⑧ ⑨ ⑩

Describe your pain / symptoms

Where do you feel it?

	am	pm
_____	☐	☐
_____	☐	☐
_____	☐	☐
_____	☐	☐
_____	☐	☐
_____	☐	☐
_____	☐	☐
_____	☐	☐

Front   *Back*

What about your...?

		Feeling sick?
Mood	① ② ③ ④ ⑤ ⑥ ⑦ ⑧ ⑨ ⑩	☐ Nope!
Energy levels	① ② ③ ④ ⑤ ⑥ ⑦ ⑧ ⑨ ⑩	☐ Yes...
Mental clarity	① ② ③ ④ ⑤ ⑥ ⑦ ⑧ ⑨ ⑩	

☐ Nausea   ☐ Diarrhea   ☐ Vomiting   ☐ Sore throat

☐ Congestion   ☐ Coughing   ☐ Chills   ☐ Fever

Other symptoms: _____

LET'S EXPLORE SOME MORE #2

Hours of Sleep ① ② ③ ④ ⑤ ⑥ ⑦ ⑧ ⑨ ⑩ ⊕
Sleep Quality ① ② ③ ④ ⑤ ⑥ ⑦ ⑧ ⑨ ⑩

WEATHER

☐ Hot   ☐ Mild   ☐ Cold   BM Pressure: _____

☐ Dry   ☐ Humid   ☐ Wet   Allergen Levels: _____

STRESS LEVELS

None	Low	Medium	High	Max	@$#%!

FOOD / MEDICATIONS

FOOD / DRINKS	MEDS / SUPPLEMENTS	TIME	DOSE
	☐ usual daily medication		

EXERCISE / DAILY ACTIVITY

☐ Damn right, I worked out.

☐ I managed to exercise a bit.

☐ No, I haven't exercised at all.

☐ I did some stuff, and that counts.

DETAILS

NOTES / TRIGGERS / IMPROVEMENTS

_____
_____
_____

WRITE ONE THING YOU'RE GRATEFUL FOR
_____

Date: _____

How are you feeling today?

Like death	Like shit	Not good	Meh	Good	Great!	Amazing!

RATE YOUR PAIN LEVEL

① ② ③ ④ ⑤ ⑥ ⑦ ⑧ ⑨ ⑩

Describe your pain / symptoms

Where do you feel it?

am	pm
☐	☐
☐	☐
☐	☐
☐	☐
☐	☐
☐	☐
☐	☐
☐	☐

Front *Back*

What about your...?

Feeling sick?

Mood ① ② ③ ④ ⑤ ⑥ ⑦ ⑧ ⑨ ⑩ ☐ Nope!

Energy levels ① ② ③ ④ ⑤ ⑥ ⑦ ⑧ ⑨ ⑩ ☐ Yes...

Mental clarity ① ② ③ ④ ⑤ ⑥ ⑦ ⑧ ⑨ ⑩

☐ Nausea ☐ Diarrhea ☐ Vomiting ☐ Sore throat

☐ Congestion ☐ Coughing ☐ Chills ☐ Fever

Other symptoms:

LET'S EXPLORE SOME MORE #3

Hours of Sleep ① ② ③ ④ ⑤ ⑥ ⑦ ⑧ ⑨ ⑩ ⊕

Sleep Quality ① ② ③ ④ ⑤ ⑥ ⑦ ⑧ ⑨ ⑩

WEATHER

☐ Hot   ☐ Mild   ☐ Cold   BM Pressure: _____

☐ Dry   ☐ Humid   ☐ Wet   Allergen Levels: _____

STRESS LEVELS

None	Low	Medium	High	Max	@$#%!

FOOD / MEDICATIONS

FOOD / DRINKS	MEDS / SUPPLEMENTS	TIME	DOSE

☐ usual daily medication

EXERCISE / DAILY ACTIVITY

☐ Damn right, I worked out.

☐ I managed to exercise a bit.

☐ No, I haven't exercised at all.

☐ I did some stuff, and that counts.

DETAILS

NOTES / TRIGGERS / IMPROVEMENTS

WRITE ONE THING YOU'RE GRATEFUL FOR

Date: _____

How are you feeling today?

Like death	Like shit	Not good	Meh	Good	Great!	Amazing!

RATE YOUR PAIN LEVEL

① ② ③ ④ ⑤ ⑥ ⑦ ⑧ ⑨ ⑩

Describe your pain / symptoms

	am	pm
_____	☐	☐
_____	☐	☐
_____	☐	☐
_____	☐	☐
_____	☐	☐
_____	☐	☐
_____	☐	☐
_____	☐	☐

Where do you feel it?

Front   *Back*

What about your...?

Mood	① ② ③ ④ ⑤ ⑥ ⑦ ⑧ ⑨ ⑩
Energy levels	① ② ③ ④ ⑤ ⑥ ⑦ ⑧ ⑨ ⑩
Mental clarity	① ② ③ ④ ⑤ ⑥ ⑦ ⑧ ⑨ ⑩

Feeling sick?

☐ Nope!

☐ Yes...

☐ Nausea ☐ Diarrhea ☐ Vomiting ☐ Sore throat

☐ Congestion ☐ Coughing ☐ Chills ☐ Fever

Other symptoms: _____

LET'S EXPLORE SOME MORE #4

Hours of Sleep ① ② ③ ④ ⑤ ⑥ ⑦ ⑧ ⑨ ⑩ ⊕

Sleep Quality ① ② ③ ④ ⑤ ⑥ ⑦ ⑧ ⑨ ⑩

WEATHER

☐ Hot ☐ Mild ☐ Cold BM Pressure: _____

☐ Dry ☐ Humid ☐ Wet Allergen Levels: _____

STRESS LEVELS

| None | Low | Medium | High | Max | @$#%! |

FOOD / MEDICATIONS

FOOD / DRINKS	MEDS / SUPPLEMENTS	TIME	DOSE
	☐ usual daily medication		

EXERCISE / DAILY ACTIVITY

☐ Damn right, I worked out.

☐ I managed to exercise a bit.

☐ No, I haven't exercised at all.

☐ I did some stuff, and that counts.

DETAILS

NOTES / TRIGGERS / IMPROVEMENTS

WRITE ONE THING YOU'RE GRATEFUL FOR

Date: _____

How are you feeling today?

| Like death | Like shit | Not good | Meh | Good | Great! | Amazing! |

RATE YOUR PAIN LEVEL

(1) (2) (3) (4) (5) (6) (7) (8) (9) (10)

Describe your pain / symptoms

	am	pm
_____	☐	☐
_____	☐	☐
_____	☐	☐
_____	☐	☐
_____	☐	☐
_____	☐	☐
_____	☐	☐
_____	☐	☐

Where do you feel it?

Front   *Back*

What about your...?

Mood	(1) (2) (3) (4) (5) (6) (7) (8) (9) (10)
Energy levels	(1) (2) (3) (4) (5) (6) (7) (8) (9) (10)
Mental clarity	(1) (2) (3) (4) (5) (6) (7) (8) (9) (10)

Feeling sick?

☐ Nope!

☐ Yes...

| ☐ Nausea | ☐ Diarrhea | ☐ Vomiting | ☐ Sore throat |
| ☐ Congestion | ☐ Coughing | ☐ Chills | ☐ Fever |

Other symptoms: _____

LET'S EXPLORE SOME MORE #5

Hours of Sleep (1)(2)(3)(4)(5)(6)(7)(8)(9)(10)(+)
Sleep Quality (1)(2)(3)(4)(5)(6)(7)(8)(9)(10)

WEATHER

☐ Hot   ☐ Mild   ☐ Cold   BM Pressure: _____

☐ Dry   ☐ Humid   ☐ Wet   Allergen Levels: _____

STRESS LEVELS

None	Low	Medium	High	Max	@$#%!

FOOD / MEDICATIONS

FOOD / DRINKS	MEDS / SUPPLEMENTS	TIME	DOSE

☐ usual daily medication

EXERCISE / DAILY ACTIVITY

☐ Damn right, I worked out.

☐ I managed to exercise a bit.

☐ No, I haven't exercised at all.

☐ I did some stuff, and that counts.

DETAILS

NOTES / TRIGGERS / IMPROVEMENTS

_____

_____

_____

WRITE ONE THING YOU'RE GRATEFUL FOR

_____

Date: _____

How are you feeling today?

Like death   Like shit   Not good   Meh   Good   Great!   Amazing!

RATE YOUR PAIN LEVEL

① ② ③ ④ ⑤ ⑥ ⑦ ⑧ ⑨ ⑩

Describe your pain / symptoms

Where do you feel it?

	am	pm
_____	☐	☐
_____	☐	☐
_____	☐	☐
_____	☐	☐
_____	☐	☐
_____	☐	☐
_____	☐	☐
_____	☐	☐

Front   *Back*

What about your...?

Feeling sick?

Mood	① ② ③ ④ ⑤ ⑥ ⑦ ⑧ ⑨ ⑩	☐ Nope!
Energy levels	① ② ③ ④ ⑤ ⑥ ⑦ ⑧ ⑨ ⑩	☐ Yes...
Mental clarity	① ② ③ ④ ⑤ ⑥ ⑦ ⑧ ⑨ ⑩	

☐ Nausea   ☐ Diarrhea   ☐ Vomiting   ☐ Sore throat

☐ Congestion   ☐ Coughing   ☐ Chills   ☐ Fever

Other symptoms: _____

LET'S EXPLORE SOME MORE #6

Hours of Sleep ① ② ③ ④ ⑤ ⑥ ⑦ ⑧ ⑨ ⑩ ⊕

Sleep Quality ① ② ③ ④ ⑤ ⑥ ⑦ ⑧ ⑨ ⑩

WEATHER

☐ Hot ☐ Mild ☐ Cold BM Pressure: _____

☐ Dry ☐ Humid ☐ Wet Allergen Levels: _____

STRESS LEVELS

None	Low	Medium	High	Max	@$#%!

FOOD / MEDICATIONS

FOOD / DRINKS	MEDS / SUPPLEMENTS	TIME	DOSE

☐ usual daily medication

EXERCISE / DAILY ACTIVITY

☐ Damn right, I worked out.

☐ I managed to exercise a bit.

☐ No, I haven't exercised at all.

☐ I did some stuff, and that counts.

DETAILS

NOTES / TRIGGERS / IMPROVEMENTS

WRITE ONE THING YOU'RE GRATEFUL FOR

Date: _____

How are you feeling today?

Like death	Like shit	Not good	Meh	Good	Great!	Amazing!

RATE YOUR PAIN LEVEL

①②③④⑤⑥⑦⑧⑨⑩

Describe your pain / symptoms

	am	pm
_____	☐	☐
_____	☐	☐
_____	☐	☐
_____	☐	☐
_____	☐	☐
_____	☐	☐
_____	☐	☐
_____	☐	☐

Where do you feel it?

Front   *Back*

What about your...?

Mood	①②③④⑤⑥⑦⑧⑨⑩
Energy levels	①②③④⑤⑥⑦⑧⑨⑩
Mental clarity	①②③④⑤⑥⑦⑧⑨⑩

Feeling sick?

☐ Nope!

☐ Yes...

☐ Nausea ☐ Diarrhea ☐ Vomiting ☐ Sore throat

☐ Congestion ☐ Coughing ☐ Chills ☐ Fever

Other symptoms: _____

Hours of Sleep ① ② ③ ④ ⑤ ⑥ ⑦ ⑧ ⑨ ⑩ ⊕
Sleep Quality ① ② ③ ④ ⑤ ⑥ ⑦ ⑧ ⑨ ⑩

WEATHER

☐ Hot ☐ Mild ☐ Cold BM Pressure: _____

☐ Dry ☐ Humid ☐ Wet Allergen Levels: _____

STRESS LEVELS

None	Low	Medium	High	Max	@$#%!

FOOD / MEDICATIONS

FOOD / DRINKS	MEDS / SUPPLEMENTS	TIME	DOSE

☐ usual daily medication

EXERCISE / DAILY ACTIVITY

☐ Damn right, I worked out.

☐ I managed to exercise a bit.

☐ No, I haven't exercised at all.

☐ I did some stuff, and that counts.

DETAILS

NOTES / TRIGGERS / IMPROVEMENTS

_____

_____

_____

WRITE ONE THING YOU'RE GRATEFUL FOR

_____

Date: _____

How are you feeling today?

Like death   Like shit   Not good   Meh   Good   Great!   Amazing!

RATE YOUR PAIN LEVEL

(1) (2) (3) (4) (5) (6) (7) (8) (9) (10)

Describe your pain / symptoms

Where do you feel it?

	am	pm
_____	☐	☐
_____	☐	☐
_____	☐	☐
_____	☐	☐
_____	☐	☐
_____	☐	☐
_____	☐	☐
_____	☐	☐

Front

Back

What about your...?

Feeling sick?

Mood   (1)(2)(3)(4)(5)(6)(7)(8)(9)(10)   ☐ Nope!

Energy levels   (1)(2)(3)(4)(5)(6)(7)(8)(9)(10)   ☐ Yes...

Mental clarity   (1)(2)(3)(4)(5)(6)(7)(8)(9)(10)

☐ Nausea   ☐ Diarrhea   ☐ Vomiting   ☐ Sore throat

☐ Congestion   ☐ Coughing   ☐ Chills   ☐ Fever

Other symptoms: _____

Hours of Sleep ① ② ③ ④ ⑤ ⑥ ⑦ ⑧ ⑨ ⑩ ⊕
Sleep Quality ① ② ③ ④ ⑤ ⑥ ⑦ ⑧ ⑨ ⑩

WEATHER

☐ Hot ☐ Mild ☐ Cold BM Pressure: _____

☐ Dry ☐ Humid ☐ Wet Allergen Levels: _____

STRESS LEVELS

| None | Low | Medium | High | Max | @$#%! |

FOOD / MEDICATIONS

FOOD / DRINKS	MEDS / SUPPLEMENTS	TIME	DOSE

☐ usual daily medication

EXERCISE / DAILY ACTIVITY

☐ Damn right, I worked out.

☐ I managed to exercise a bit.

☐ No, I haven't exercised at all.

☐ I did some stuff, and that counts.

DETAILS

NOTES / TRIGGERS / IMPROVEMENTS

WRITE ONE THING YOU'RE GRATEFUL FOR

Date: _____

How are you feeling today?

Like death   Like shit   Not good   Meh   Good   Great!   Amazing!

RATE YOUR PAIN LEVEL

① ② ③ ④ ⑤ ⑥ ⑦ ⑧ ⑨ ⑩

Describe your pain / symptoms

	am	pm
	☐	☐
	☐	☐
	☐	☐
	☐	☐
	☐	☐
	☐	☐
	☐	☐
	☐	☐

Where do you feel it?

Front   *Back*

What about your...?

Mood	① ② ③ ④ ⑤ ⑥ ⑦ ⑧ ⑨ ⑩
Energy levels	① ② ③ ④ ⑤ ⑥ ⑦ ⑧ ⑨ ⑩
Mental clarity	① ② ③ ④ ⑤ ⑥ ⑦ ⑧ ⑨ ⑩

Feeling sick?

☐ Nope!

☐ Yes...

☐ Nausea   ☐ Diarrhea   ☐ Vomiting   ☐ Sore throat

☐ Congestion   ☐ Coughing   ☐ Chills   ☐ Fever

Other symptoms: _____

Hours of Sleep ① ② ③ ④ ⑤ ⑥ ⑦ ⑧ ⑨ ⑩ ⊕

Sleep Quality ① ② ③ ④ ⑤ ⑥ ⑦ ⑧ ⑨ ⑩

WEATHER

☐ Hot ☐ Mild ☐ Cold BM Pressure: _____

☐ Dry ☐ Humid ☐ Wet Allergen Levels: _____

STRESS LEVELS

None	Low	Medium	High	Max	@$#%!

FOOD / MEDICATIONS

FOOD / DRINKS	MEDS / SUPPLEMENTS	TIME	DOSE

☐ usual daily medication

EXERCISE / DAILY ACTIVITY

☐ Damn right, I worked out.

☐ I managed to exercise a bit.

☐ No, I haven't exercised at all.

☐ I did some stuff, and that counts.

DETAILS

NOTES / TRIGGERS / IMPROVEMENTS

_____

_____

_____

WRITE ONE THING YOU'RE GRATEFUL FOR

_____

Date: _____

How are you feeling today?

Like death	Like shit	Not good	Meh	Good	Great!	Amazing!

RATE YOUR PAIN LEVEL

① ② ③ ④ ⑤ ⑥ ⑦ ⑧ ⑨ ⑩

Describe your pain / symptoms   Where do you feel it?

	am	pm	Front	Back
	☐	☐		
	☐	☐		
	☐	☐		
	☐	☐		
	☐	☐		
	☐	☐		
	☐	☐		
	☐	☐		

What about your...?   Feeling sick?

Mood   ① ② ③ ④ ⑤ ⑥ ⑦ ⑧ ⑨ ⑩   ☐ Nope!

Energy levels   ① ② ③ ④ ⑤ ⑥ ⑦ ⑧ ⑨ ⑩   ☐ Yes...

Mental clarity ① ② ③ ④ ⑤ ⑥ ⑦ ⑧ ⑨ ⑩

☐ Nausea   ☐ Diarrhea   ☐ Vomiting   ☐ Sore throat

☐ Congestion ☐ Coughing   ☐ Chills   ☐ Fever

Other symptoms: _____

LET'S EXPLORE SOME MORE

Hours of Sleep ① ② ③ ④ ⑤ ⑥ ⑦ ⑧ ⑨ ⑩ ⊕

Sleep Quality ① ② ③ ④ ⑤ ⑥ ⑦ ⑧ ⑨ ⑩

WEATHER

☐ Hot ☐ Mild ☐ Cold BM Pressure: _____

☐ Dry ☐ Humid ☐ Wet Allergen Levels: _____

STRESS LEVELS

None	Low	Medium	High	Max	@$#%!

FOOD / MEDICATIONS

FOOD / DRINKS	MEDS / SUPPLEMENTS	TIME	DOSE

☐ usual daily medication

EXERCISE / DAILY ACTIVITY

☐ Damn right, I worked out.

☐ I managed to exercise a bit.

☐ No, I haven't exercised at all.

☐ I did some stuff, and that counts.

DETAILS

NOTES / TRIGGERS / IMPROVEMENTS

_____

_____

_____

WRITE ONE THING YOU'RE GRATEFUL FOR

_____

Date: _____

How are you feeling today?

Like death	Like shit	Not good	Meh	Good	Great!	Amazing!

RATE YOUR PAIN LEVEL

① ② ③ ④ ⑤ ⑥ ⑦ ⑧ ⑨ ⑩

Describe your pain / symptoms

	am	pm
_____	☐	☐
_____	☐	☐
_____	☐	☐
_____	☐	☐
_____	☐	☐
_____	☐	☐
_____	☐	☐
_____	☐	☐

Where do you feel it?

Front   *Back*

What about your...?

Mood	① ② ③ ④ ⑤ ⑥ ⑦ ⑧ ⑨ ⑩
Energy levels	① ② ③ ④ ⑤ ⑥ ⑦ ⑧ ⑨ ⑩
Mental clarity	① ② ③ ④ ⑤ ⑥ ⑦ ⑧ ⑨ ⑩

Feeling sick?

☐ Nope!

☐ Yes...

☐ Nausea ☐ Diarrhea ☐ Vomiting ☐ Sore throat

☐ Congestion ☐ Coughing ☐ Chills ☐ Fever

Other symptoms: _____

LET'S EXPLORE SOME MORE #11

Hours of Sleep ① ② ③ ④ ⑤ ⑥ ⑦ ⑧ ⑨ ⑩ ⊕
Sleep Quality ① ② ③ ④ ⑤ ⑥ ⑦ ⑧ ⑨ ⑩

WEATHER

☐ Hot ☐ Mild ☐ Cold BM Pressure: _____

☐ Dry ☐ Humid ☐ Wet Allergen Levels: _____

STRESS LEVELS

None	Low	Medium	High	Max	@$#%!

FOOD / MEDICATIONS

FOOD / DRINKS	MEDS / SUPPLEMENTS	TIME	DOSE

☐ usual daily medication

EXERCISE / DAILY ACTIVITY

DETAILS

☐ Damn right, I worked out.

☐ I managed to exercise a bit.

☐ No, I haven't exercised at all.

☐ I did some stuff, and that counts.

NOTES / TRIGGERS / IMPROVEMENTS

WRITE ONE THING YOU'RE GRATEFUL FOR

Date: _____

How are you feeling today?

Like death	Like shit	Not good	Meh	Good	Great!	Amazing!

RATE YOUR PAIN LEVEL

① ② ③ ④ ⑤ ⑥ ⑦ ⑧ ⑨ ⑩

Describe your pain / symptoms

	am	pm
_____	☐	☐
_____	☐	☐
_____	☐	☐
_____	☐	☐
_____	☐	☐
_____	☐	☐
_____	☐	☐
_____	☐	☐

Where do you feel it?

Front   *Back*

What about your...?

Mood	① ② ③ ④ ⑤ ⑥ ⑦ ⑧ ⑨ ⑩
Energy levels	① ② ③ ④ ⑤ ⑥ ⑦ ⑧ ⑨ ⑩
Mental clarity	① ② ③ ④ ⑤ ⑥ ⑦ ⑧ ⑨ ⑩

Feeling sick?

☐ Nope!
☐ Yes...

☐ Nausea   ☐ Diarrhea   ☐ Vomiting   ☐ Sore throat
☐ Congestion ☐ Coughing   ☐ Chills   ☐ Fever

Other symptoms: _____

LET'S EXPLORE SOME MORE

Hours of Sleep (1) (2) (3) (4) (5) (6) (7) (8) (9) (10) (+)

Sleep Quality (1) (2) (3) (4) (5) (6) (7) (8) (9) (10)

WEATHER

☐ Hot ☐ Mild ☐ Cold BM Pressure: _____

☐ Dry ☐ Humid ☐ Wet Allergen Levels: _____

STRESS LEVELS

None	Low	Medium	High	Max	@$#%!

FOOD / MEDICATIONS

FOOD / DRINKS	MEDS / SUPPLEMENTS	TIME	DOSE

☐ usual daily medication

EXERCISE / DAILY ACTIVITY

DETAILS

☐ Damn right, I worked out.

☐ I managed to exercise a bit.

☐ No, I haven't exercised at all.

☐ I did some stuff, and that counts.

NOTES / TRIGGERS / IMPROVEMENTS

WRITE ONE THING YOU'RE GRATEFUL FOR

Date: _____

How are you feeling today?

| Like death | Like shit | Not good | Meh | Good | Great! | Amazing! |

RATE YOUR PAIN LEVEL

① ② ③ ④ ⑤ ⑥ ⑦ ⑧ ⑨ ⑩

Describe your pain / symptoms   **Where do you feel it?**

	am	pm
	☐	☐
	☐	☐
	☐	☐
	☐	☐
	☐	☐
	☐	☐
	☐	☐
	☐	☐

Front   *Back*

What about your...?   Feeling sick?

Mood   ① ② ③ ④ ⑤ ⑥ ⑦ ⑧ ⑨ ⑩   ☐ Nope!

Energy levels   ① ② ③ ④ ⑤ ⑥ ⑦ ⑧ ⑨ ⑩   ☐ Yes...

Mental clarity ① ② ③ ④ ⑤ ⑥ ⑦ ⑧ ⑨ ⑩

☐ Nausea   ☐ Diarrhea   ☐ Vomiting   ☐ Sore throat

☐ Congestion   ☐ Coughing   ☐ Chills   ☐ Fever

Other symptoms: _____

LET'S EXPLORE SOME MORE #13

Hours of Sleep ① ② ③ ④ ⑤ ⑥ ⑦ ⑧ ⑨ ⑩ ⊕

Sleep Quality ① ② ③ ④ ⑤ ⑥ ⑦ ⑧ ⑨ ⑩

WEATHER

☐ Hot ☐ Mild ☐ Cold BM Pressure: _____

☐ Dry ☐ Humid ☐ Wet Allergen Levels: _____

STRESS LEVELS

None	Low	Medium	High	Max	@$#%!

FOOD / MEDICATIONS

FOOD / DRINKS	MEDS / SUPPLEMENTS	TIME	DOSE

☐ usual daily medication

EXERCISE / DAILY ACTIVITY

☐ Damn right, I worked out.

☐ I managed to exercise a bit.

☐ No, I haven't exercised at all.

☐ I did some stuff, and that counts.

DETAILS

NOTES / TRIGGERS / IMPROVEMENTS

_____

_____

_____

WRITE ONE THING YOU'RE GRATEFUL FOR

_____

Date:_____

How are you feeling today?

Like death	Like shit	Not good	Meh	Good	Great!	Amazing!

RATE YOUR PAIN LEVEL

① ② ③ ④ ⑤ ⑥ ⑦ ⑧ ⑨ ⑩

Describe your pain / symptoms

	am	pm
	☐	☐
	☐	☐
	☐	☐
	☐	☐
	☐	☐
	☐	☐
	☐	☐
	☐	☐

Where do you feel it?

Front   *Back*

What about your...?

Mood	① ② ③ ④ ⑤ ⑥ ⑦ ⑧ ⑨ ⑩
Energy levels	① ② ③ ④ ⑤ ⑥ ⑦ ⑧ ⑨ ⑩
Mental clarity	① ② ③ ④ ⑤ ⑥ ⑦ ⑧ ⑨ ⑩

Feeling sick?

☐ Nope!
☐ Yes...

☐ Nausea   ☐ Diarrhea   ☐ Vomiting   ☐ Sore throat
☐ Congestion   ☐ Coughing   ☐ Chills   ☐ Fever

Other symptoms:_____

LET'S EXPLORE SOME MORE #14

Hours of Sleep ① ② ③ ④ ⑤ ⑥ ⑦ ⑧ ⑨ ⑩ ⊕
Sleep Quality ① ② ③ ④ ⑤ ⑥ ⑦ ⑧ ⑨ ⑩

WEATHER

☐ Hot ☐ Mild ☐ Cold BM Pressure: _____
☐ Dry ☐ Humid ☐ Wet Allergen Levels: _____

STRESS LEVELS

None	Low	Medium	High	Max	@$#%!

FOOD / MEDICATIONS

FOOD / DRINKS	MEDS / SUPPLEMENTS	TIME	DOSE

☐ usual daily medication

EXERCISE / DAILY ACTIVITY

DETAILS

☐ Damn right, I worked out.
☐ I managed to exercise a bit.
☐ No, I haven't exercised at all.
☐ I did some stuff, and that counts.

NOTES / TRIGGERS / IMPROVEMENTS

WRITE ONE THING YOU'RE GRATEFUL FOR

Date: _____

How are you feeling today?

Like death	Like shit	Not good	Meh	Good	Great!	Amazing!

RATE YOUR PAIN LEVEL

① ② ③ ④ ⑤ ⑥ ⑦ ⑧ ⑨ ⑩

Describe your pain / symptoms

	am	pm
_____	☐	☐
_____	☐	☐
_____	☐	☐
_____	☐	☐
_____	☐	☐
_____	☐	☐
_____	☐	☐
_____	☐	☐

Where do you feel it?

Front   *Back*

What about your...?

Mood	① ② ③ ④ ⑤ ⑥ ⑦ ⑧ ⑨ ⑩
Energy levels	① ② ③ ④ ⑤ ⑥ ⑦ ⑧ ⑨ ⑩
Mental clarity	① ② ③ ④ ⑤ ⑥ ⑦ ⑧ ⑨ ⑩

Feeling sick?

☐ Nope!

☐ Yes...

☐ Nausea   ☐ Diarrhea   ☐ Vomiting   ☐ Sore throat

☐ Congestion   ☐ Coughing   ☐ Chills   ☐ Fever

Other symptoms: _____

LET'S EXPLORE SOME MORE #15

Hours of Sleep   ① ② ③ ④ ⑤ ⑥ ⑦ ⑧ ⑨ ⑩ ⊕

Sleep Quality   ① ② ③ ④ ⑤ ⑥ ⑦ ⑧ ⑨ ⑩

WEATHER

☐ Hot   ☐ Mild   ☐ Cold   BM Pressure: _____

☐ Dry   ☐ Humid   ☐ Wet   Allergen Levels: _____

STRESS LEVELS

None	Low	Medium	High	Max	@$#%!

FOOD / MEDICATIONS

FOOD / DRINKS	MEDS / SUPPLEMENTS	TIME	DOSE

☐ usual daily medication

EXERCISE / DAILY ACTIVITY

☐ Damn right, I worked out.

☐ I managed to exercise a bit.

☐ No, I haven't exercised at all.

☐ I did some stuff, and that counts.

DETAILS

NOTES / TRIGGERS / IMPROVEMENTS

_____

_____

WRITE ONE THING YOU'RE GRATEFUL FOR

_____

Date: _____

How are you feeling today?

Like death	Like shit	Not good	Meh	Good	Great!	Amazing!

RATE YOUR PAIN LEVEL

① ② ③ ④ ⑤ ⑥ ⑦ ⑧ ⑨ ⑩

Describe your pain / symptoms

	am	pm
_____	☐	☐
_____	☐	☐
_____	☐	☐
_____	☐	☐
_____	☐	☐
_____	☐	☐
_____	☐	☐
_____	☐	☐

Where do you feel it?

Front *Back*

What about your...?

Mood	① ② ③ ④ ⑤ ⑥ ⑦ ⑧ ⑨ ⑩
Energy levels	① ② ③ ④ ⑤ ⑥ ⑦ ⑧ ⑨ ⑩
Mental clarity	① ② ③ ④ ⑤ ⑥ ⑦ ⑧ ⑨ ⑩

Feeling sick?

☐ Nope!

☐ Yes...

☐ Nausea ☐ Diarrhea ☐ Vomiting ☐ Sore throat

☐ Congestion ☐ Coughing ☐ Chills ☐ Fever

Other symptoms: _____

LET'S EXPLORE SOME MORE #16

Hours of Sleep ① ② ③ ④ ⑤ ⑥ ⑦ ⑧ ⑨ ⑩ ⊕

Sleep Quality ① ② ③ ④ ⑤ ⑥ ⑦ ⑧ ⑨ ⑩

WEATHER

☐ Hot ☐ Mild ☐ Cold BM Pressure: _____

☐ Dry ☐ Humid ☐ Wet Allergen Levels: _____

STRESS LEVELS

None	Low	Medium	High	Max	@$#%!

FOOD / MEDICATIONS

FOOD / DRINKS	MEDS / SUPPLEMENTS	TIME	DOSE
	☐ usual daily medication		

EXERCISE / DAILY ACTIVITY

☐ Damn right, I worked out.

☐ I managed to exercise a bit.

☐ No, I haven't exercised at all.

☐ I did some stuff, and that counts.

DETAILS

NOTES / TRIGGERS / IMPROVEMENTS

WRITE ONE THING YOU'RE GRATEFUL FOR

Date: _____

How are you feeling today?

Like death	Like shit	Not good	Meh	Good	Great!	Amazing!

RATE YOUR PAIN LEVEL

① ② ③ ④ ⑤ ⑥ ⑦ ⑧ ⑨ ⑩

Describe your pain / symptoms

	am	pm
_____	☐	☐
_____	☐	☐
_____	☐	☐
_____	☐	☐
_____	☐	☐
_____	☐	☐
_____	☐	☐
_____	☐	☐

Where do you feel it?

Front   *Back*

What about your...?

Mood	① ② ③ ④ ⑤ ⑥ ⑦ ⑧ ⑨ ⑩
Energy levels	① ② ③ ④ ⑤ ⑥ ⑦ ⑧ ⑨ ⑩
Mental clarity	① ② ③ ④ ⑤ ⑥ ⑦ ⑧ ⑨ ⑩

Feeling sick?

☐ Nope!

☐ Yes...

☐ Nausea   ☐ Diarrhea   ☐ Vomiting   ☐ Sore throat

☐ Congestion   ☐ Coughing   ☐ Chills   ☐ Fever

Other symptoms: _____

LET'S EXPLORE SOME MORE #17

Hours of Sleep ① ② ③ ④ ⑤ ⑥ ⑦ ⑧ ⑨ ⑩ ⊕

Sleep Quality ① ② ③ ④ ⑤ ⑥ ⑦ ⑧ ⑨ ⑩

WEATHER

☐ Hot   ☐ Mild   ☐ Cold   BM Pressure: _____

☐ Dry   ☐ Humid   ☐ Wet   Allergen Levels: _____

STRESS LEVELS

None	Low	Medium	High	Max	@$#%!

FOOD / MEDICATIONS

FOOD / DRINKS	MEDS / SUPPLEMENTS	TIME	DOSE

☐ usual daily medication

EXERCISE / DAILY ACTIVITY

☐ Damn right, I worked out.

☐ I managed to exercise a bit.

☐ No, I haven't exercised at all.

☐ I did some stuff, and that counts.

DETAILS

NOTES / TRIGGERS / IMPROVEMENTS

WRITE ONE THING YOU'RE GRATEFUL FOR

Date: _____

How are you feeling today?

Like death   Like shit   Not good   Meh   Good   Great!   Amazing!

RATE YOUR PAIN LEVEL

① ② ③ ④ ⑤ ⑥ ⑦ ⑧ ⑨ ⑩

Describe your pain / symptoms

	am	pm
_____	☐	☐
_____	☐	☐
_____	☐	☐
_____	☐	☐
_____	☐	☐
_____	☐	☐
_____	☐	☐
	☐	☐

Where do you feel it?

Front   *Back*

What about your...?

Mood	①	②	③	④	⑤	⑥	⑦	⑧	⑨	⑩	
Energy levels	①	②	③	④	⑤	⑥	⑦	⑧	⑨	⑩	
Mental clarity	①	②	③	④	⑤	⑥	⑦	⑧	⑨	⑩	

Feeling sick?

☐ Nope!

☐ Yes...

☐ Nausea   ☐ Diarrhea   ☐ Vomiting   ☐ Sore throat

☐ Congestion   ☐ Coughing   ☐ Chills   ☐ Fever

Other symptoms: _____

LET'S EXPLORE SOME MORE #18

Hours of Sleep ① ② ③ ④ ⑤ ⑥ ⑦ ⑧ ⑨ ⑩ ⊕
Sleep Quality ① ② ③ ④ ⑤ ⑥ ⑦ ⑧ ⑨ ⑩

WEATHER

☐ Hot ☐ Mild ☐ Cold BM Pressure: _____

☐ Dry ☐ Humid ☐ Wet Allergen Levels: _____

STRESS LEVELS

None	Low	Medium	High	Max	@$#%!

FOOD / MEDICATIONS

FOOD / DRINKS	MEDS / SUPPLEMENTS	TIME	DOSE
	☐ usual daily medication		

EXERCISE / DAILY ACTIVITY

☐ Damn right, I worked out.

☐ I managed to exercise a bit.

☐ No, I haven't exercised at all.

☐ I did some stuff, and that counts.

DETAILS

NOTES / TRIGGERS / IMPROVEMENTS

_____

_____

_____

WRITE ONE THING YOU'RE GRATEFUL FOR

_____

Date: _____

How are you feeling today?

Like death   Like shit   Not good   Meh   Good   Great!   Amazing!

RATE YOUR PAIN LEVEL

① ② ③ ④ ⑤ ⑥ ⑦ ⑧ ⑨ ⑩

Describe your pain / symptoms

	am	pm
	☐	☐
	☐	☐
	☐	☐
	☐	☐
	☐	☐
	☐	☐
	☐	☐
	☐	☐

Where do you feel it?

Front   *Back*

What about your...?

Mood	①	②	③	④	⑤	⑥	⑦	⑧	⑨	⑩
Energy levels	①	②	③	④	⑤	⑥	⑦	⑧	⑨	⑩
Mental clarity	①	②	③	④	⑤	⑥	⑦	⑧	⑨	⑩

Feeling sick?

☐ Nope!

☐ Yes...

☐ Nausea   ☐ Diarrhea   ☐ Vomiting   ☐ Sore throat

☐ Congestion   ☐ Coughing   ☐ Chills   ☐ Fever

Other symptoms:

LET'S EXPLORE SOME MORE #19

Hours of Sleep ① ② ③ ④ ⑤ ⑥ ⑦ ⑧ ⑨ ⑩ ⊕

Sleep Quality ① ② ③ ④ ⑤ ⑥ ⑦ ⑧ ⑨ ⑩

WEATHER

☐ Hot ☐ Mild ☐ Cold BM Pressure: _____

☐ Dry ☐ Humid ☐ Wet Allergen Levels: _____

STRESS LEVELS

| None | Low | Medium | High | Max | @$#%! |

FOOD / MEDICATIONS

FOOD / DRINKS	MEDS / SUPPLEMENTS	TIME	DOSE

☐ usual daily medication

EXERCISE / DAILY ACTIVITY

DETAILS

☐ Damn right, I worked out.

☐ I managed to exercise a bit.

☐ No, I haven't exercised at all.

☐ I did some stuff, and that counts.

NOTES / TRIGGERS / IMPROVEMENTS

WRITE ONE THING YOU'RE GRATEFUL FOR

Date: _____

How are you feeling today?

Like death	Like shit	Not good	Meh	Good	Great!	Amazing!

RATE YOUR PAIN LEVEL

① ② ③ ④ ⑤ ⑥ ⑦ ⑧ ⑨ ⑩

Describe your pain / symptoms

	am	pm
_____	☐	☐
_____	☐	☐
_____	☐	☐
_____	☐	☐
_____	☐	☐
_____	☐	☐
_____	☐	☐
_____	☐	☐

Where do you feel it?

Front　　*Back*

What about your...?

Mood	① ② ③ ④ ⑤ ⑥ ⑦ ⑧ ⑨ ⑩
Energy levels	① ② ③ ④ ⑤ ⑥ ⑦ ⑧ ⑨ ⑩
Mental clarity	① ② ③ ④ ⑤ ⑥ ⑦ ⑧ ⑨ ⑩

Feeling sick?

☐ Nope!
☐ Yes...

☐ Nausea　　☐ Diarrhea　　☐ Vomiting　　☐ Sore throat
☐ Congestion　☐ Coughing　　☐ Chills　　☐ Fever

Other symptoms: _____

LET'S EXPLORE SOME MORE #20

Hours of Sleep ① ② ③ ④ ⑤ ⑥ ⑦ ⑧ ⑨ ⑩ ⊕

Sleep Quality ① ② ③ ④ ⑤ ⑥ ⑦ ⑧ ⑨ ⑩

WEATHER

☐ Hot ☐ Mild ☐ Cold BM Pressure: _____

☐ Dry ☐ Humid ☐ Wet Allergen Levels: _____

STRESS LEVELS

None	Low	Medium	High	Max	@$#%!

FOOD / MEDICATIONS

FOOD / DRINKS	MEDS / SUPPLEMENTS	TIME	DOSE

☐ usual daily medication

EXERCISE / DAILY ACTIVITY

DETAILS

☐ Damn right, I worked out.

☐ I managed to exercise a bit.

☐ No, I haven't exercised at all.

☐ I did some stuff, and that counts.

NOTES / TRIGGERS / IMPROVEMENTS

WRITE ONE THING YOU'RE GRATEFUL FOR

Date: _____

How are you feeling today?

Like death	Like shit	Not good	Meh	Good	Great!	Amazing!

RATE YOUR PAIN LEVEL

① ② ③ ④ ⑤ ⑥ ⑦ ⑧ ⑨ ⑩

Describe your pain / symptoms

	am	pm
_____	☐	☐
_____	☐	☐
_____	☐	☐
_____	☐	☐
_____	☐	☐
_____	☐	☐
_____	☐	☐
_____	☐	☐

Where do you feel it?

Front   *Back*

What about your...?

Mood	① ② ③ ④ ⑤ ⑥ ⑦ ⑧ ⑨ ⑩
Energy levels	① ② ③ ④ ⑤ ⑥ ⑦ ⑧ ⑨ ⑩
Mental clarity	① ② ③ ④ ⑤ ⑥ ⑦ ⑧ ⑨ ⑩

Feeling sick?

☐ Nope!

☐ Yes...

☐ Nausea   ☐ Diarrhea   ☐ Vomiting   ☐ Sore throat

☐ Congestion   ☐ Coughing   ☐ Chills   ☐ Fever

Other symptoms: _____

LET'S EXPLORE SOME MORE #21

Hours of Sleep ① ② ③ ④ ⑤ ⑥ ⑦ ⑧ ⑨ ⑩ ⊕
Sleep Quality ① ② ③ ④ ⑤ ⑥ ⑦ ⑧ ⑨ ⑩

WEATHER

☐ Hot ☐ Mild ☐ Cold BM Pressure: _____
☐ Dry ☐ Humid ☐ Wet Allergen Levels: _____

STRESS LEVELS

None	Low	Medium	High	Max	@$#%!

FOOD / MEDICATIONS

FOOD / DRINKS	MEDS / SUPPLEMENTS	TIME	DOSE

☐ usual daily medication

EXERCISE / DAILY ACTIVITY

☐ Damn right, I worked out.
☐ I managed to exercise a bit.
☐ No, I haven't exercised at all.
☐ I did some stuff, and that counts.

DETAILS

NOTES / TRIGGERS / IMPROVEMENTS

WRITE ONE THING YOU'RE GRATEFUL FOR

Date: _____

How are you feeling today?

Like death	Like shit	Not good	Meh	Good	Great!	Amazing!

RATE YOUR PAIN LEVEL

① ② ③ ④ ⑤ ⑥ ⑦ ⑧ ⑨ ⑩

Describe your pain / symptoms

	am	pm
_____	☐	☐
_____	☐	☐
_____	☐	☐
_____	☐	☐
_____	☐	☐
_____	☐	☐
_____	☐	☐
_____	☐	☐

Where do you feel it?

Front   *Back*

What about your...?

Mood	① ② ③ ④ ⑤ ⑥ ⑦ ⑧ ⑨ ⑩
Energy levels	① ② ③ ④ ⑤ ⑥ ⑦ ⑧ ⑨ ⑩
Mental clarity	① ② ③ ④ ⑤ ⑥ ⑦ ⑧ ⑨ ⑩

Feeling sick?

☐ Nope!

☐ Yes...

☐ Nausea   ☐ Diarrhea   ☐ Vomiting   ☐ Sore throat

☐ Congestion   ☐ Coughing   ☐ Chills   ☐ Fever

Other symptoms: _____

LET'S EXPLORE SOME MORE #22

Hours of Sleep ① ② ③ ④ ⑤ ⑥ ⑦ ⑧ ⑨ ⑩ ⊕

Sleep Quality ① ② ③ ④ ⑤ ⑥ ⑦ ⑧ ⑨ ⑩

WEATHER

☐ Hot   ☐ Mild   ☐ Cold   BM Pressure: _____

☐ Dry   ☐ Humid   ☐ Wet   Allergen Levels: _____

STRESS LEVELS

None	Low	Medium	High	Max	@$#%!

FOOD / MEDICATIONS

FOOD / DRINKS	MEDS / SUPPLEMENTS	TIME	DOSE

☐ usual daily medication

EXERCISE / DAILY ACTIVITY

☐ Damn right, I worked out.

☐ I managed to exercise a bit.

☐ No, I haven't exercised at all.

☐ I did some stuff, and that counts.

DETAILS

NOTES / TRIGGERS / IMPROVEMENTS

WRITE ONE THING YOU'RE GRATEFUL FOR

Date: _____

How are you feeling today?

Like death	Like shit	Not good	Meh	Good	Great!	Amazing!

RATE YOUR PAIN LEVEL

(1) (2) (3) (4) (5) (6) (7) (8) (9) (10)

Describe your pain / symptoms

	am	pm
	☐	☐
	☐	☐
	☐	☐
	☐	☐
	☐	☐
	☐	☐
	☐	☐
	☐	☐

Where do you feel it?

Front   Back

What about your...?

Mood	① ② ③ ④ ⑤ ⑥ ⑦ ⑧ ⑨ ⑩
Energy levels	① ② ③ ④ ⑤ ⑥ ⑦ ⑧ ⑨ ⑩
Mental clarity	① ② ③ ④ ⑤ ⑥ ⑦ ⑧ ⑨ ⑩

Feeling sick?

☐ Nope!

☐ Yes...

☐ Nausea   ☐ Diarrhea   ☐ Vomiting   ☐ Sore throat

☐ Congestion   ☐ Coughing   ☐ Chills   ☐ Fever

Other symptoms: _____

Hours of Sleep ① ② ③ ④ ⑤ ⑥ ⑦ ⑧ ⑨ ⑩ ⊕
Sleep Quality   ① ② ③ ④ ⑤ ⑥ ⑦ ⑧ ⑨ ⑩

WEATHER

☐ Hot   ☐ Mild   ☐ Cold   BM Pressure: _____
☐ Dry   ☐ Humid   ☐ Wet   Allergen Levels: _____

STRESS LEVELS

None	Low	Medium	High	Max	@$#%!

FOOD / MEDICATIONS

FOOD / DRINKS	MEDS / SUPPLEMENTS	TIME	DOSE

☐ usual daily medication

EXERCISE / DAILY ACTIVITY

☐ Damn right, I worked out.
☐ I managed to exercise a bit.
☐ No, I haven't exercised at all.
☐ I did some stuff, and that counts.

DETAILS

NOTES / TRIGGERS / IMPROVEMENTS

_____
_____
_____

WRITE ONE THING YOU'RE GRATEFUL FOR
_____

Date: _____

How are you feeling today?

Like death	Like shit	Not good	Meh	Good	Great!	Amazing!

RATE YOUR PAIN LEVEL

① ② ③ ④ ⑤ ⑥ ⑦ ⑧ ⑨ ⑩

Describe your pain / symptoms

Where do you feel it?

	am	pm
	☐	☐
	☐	☐
	☐	☐
	☐	☐
	☐	☐
	☐	☐
	☐	☐
	☐	☐

Front　　　*Back*

What about your...?

Feeling sick?

Mood	① ② ③ ④ ⑤ ⑥ ⑦ ⑧ ⑨ ⑩
Energy levels	① ② ③ ④ ⑤ ⑥ ⑦ ⑧ ⑨ ⑩
Mental clarity	① ② ③ ④ ⑤ ⑥ ⑦ ⑧ ⑨ ⑩

☐ Nope!

☐ Yes...

☐ Nausea　　☐ Diarrhea　　☐ Vomiting　　☐ Sore throat

☐ Congestion　☐ Coughing　　☐ Chills　　☐ Fever

Other symptoms:

LET'S EXPLORE SOME MORE #24

Hours of Sleep ① ② ③ ④ ⑤ ⑥ ⑦ ⑧ ⑨ ⑩ ⊕

Sleep Quality ① ② ③ ④ ⑤ ⑥ ⑦ ⑧ ⑨ ⑩

WEATHER

☐ Hot   ☐ Mild   ☐ Cold   BM Pressure: _____

☐ Dry   ☐ Humid   ☐ Wet   Allergen Levels: _____

STRESS LEVELS

None	Low	Medium	High	Max	@$#%!

FOOD / MEDICATIONS

FOOD / DRINKS	MEDS / SUPPLEMENTS	TIME	DOSE

☐ usual daily medication

EXERCISE / DAILY ACTIVITY

☐ Damn right, I worked out.

☐ I managed to exercise a bit.

☐ No, I haven't exercised at all.

☐ I did some stuff, and that counts.

DETAILS

NOTES / TRIGGERS / IMPROVEMENTS

WRITE ONE THING YOU'RE GRATEFUL FOR

Date: _____

How are you feeling today?

Like death	Like shit	Not good	Meh	Good	Great!	Amazing!

RATE YOUR PAIN LEVEL

(1) (2) (3) (4) (5) (6) (7) (8) (9) (10)

Describe your pain / symptoms

	am	pm
_____	☐	☐
_____	☐	☐
_____	☐	☐
_____	☐	☐
_____	☐	☐
_____	☐	☐
_____	☐	☐
_____	☐	☐

Where do you feel it?

Front   *Back*

What about your...?

Mood	(1) (2) (3) (4) (5) (6) (7) (8) (9) (10)
Energy levels	(1) (2) (3) (4) (5) (6) (7) (8) (9) (10)
Mental clarity	(1) (2) (3) (4) (5) (6) (7) (8) (9) (10)

Feeling sick?

☐ Nope!
☐ Yes...

☐ Nausea   ☐ Diarrhea   ☐ Vomiting   ☐ Sore throat
☐ Congestion   ☐ Coughing   ☐ Chills   ☐ Fever

Other symptoms: _____

LET'S EXPLORE SOME MORE #25

Hours of Sleep ① ② ③ ④ ⑤ ⑥ ⑦ ⑧ ⑨ ⑩ ⊕

Sleep Quality ① ② ③ ④ ⑤ ⑥ ⑦ ⑧ ⑨ ⑩

WEATHER

☐ Hot ☐ Mild ☐ Cold BM Pressure: _____

☐ Dry ☐ Humid ☐ Wet Allergen Levels: _____

STRESS LEVELS

None	Low	Medium	High	Max	@$#%!

FOOD / MEDICATIONS

FOOD / DRINKS	MEDS / SUPPLEMENTS	TIME	DOSE

☐ usual daily medication

EXERCISE / DAILY ACTIVITY

☐ Damn right, I worked out.

☐ I managed to exercise a bit.

☐ No, I haven't exercised at all.

☐ I did some stuff, and that counts.

DETAILS

NOTES / TRIGGERS / IMPROVEMENTS

WRITE ONE THING YOU'RE GRATEFUL FOR

Date: _____

How are you feeling today?

Like death	Like shit	Not good	Meh	Good	Great!	Amazing!

RATE YOUR PAIN LEVEL

① ② ③ ④ ⑤ ⑥ ⑦ ⑧ ⑨ ⑩

Describe your pain / symptoms

	am	pm
_____	☐	☐
_____	☐	☐
_____	☐	☐
_____	☐	☐
_____	☐	☐
_____	☐	☐
_____	☐	☐
_____	☐	☐

Where do you feel it?

Front   Back

What about your...?

Mood	① ② ③ ④ ⑤ ⑥ ⑦ ⑧ ⑨ ⑩
Energy levels	① ② ③ ④ ⑤ ⑥ ⑦ ⑧ ⑨ ⑩
Mental clarity	① ② ③ ④ ⑤ ⑥ ⑦ ⑧ ⑨ ⑩

Feeling sick?

☐ Nope!
☐ Yes...

☐ Nausea   ☐ Diarrhea   ☐ Vomiting   ☐ Sore throat

☐ Congestion   ☐ Coughing   ☐ Chills   ☐ Fever

Other symptoms: _____

LET'S EXPLORE SOME MORE #26

Hours of Sleep (1)(2)(3)(4)(5)(6)(7)(8)(9)(10)(+)

Sleep Quality (1)(2)(3)(4)(5)(6)(7)(8)(9)(10)

WEATHER

☐ Hot   ☐ Mild   ☐ Cold   BM Pressure: _____

☐ Dry   ☐ Humid   ☐ Wet   Allergen Levels: _____

STRESS LEVELS

None	Low	Medium	High	Max	@$#%!

FOOD / MEDICATIONS

FOOD / DRINKS	MEDS / SUPPLEMENTS	TIME	DOSE
	☐ usual daily medication		

EXERCISE / DAILY ACTIVITY

☐ Damn right, I worked out.

☐ I managed to exercise a bit.

☐ No, I haven't exercised at all.

☐ I did some stuff, and that counts.

DETAILS

NOTES / TRIGGERS / IMPROVEMENTS

WRITE ONE THING YOU'RE GRATEFUL FOR

Date: _____

How are you feeling today?

Like death   Like shit   Not good   Meh   Good   Great!   Amazing!

RATE YOUR PAIN LEVEL

① ② ③ ④ ⑤ ⑥ ⑦ ⑧ ⑨ ⑩

Describe your pain / symptoms   **Where do you feel it?**

	am	pm
_____	☐	☐
_____	☐	☐
_____	☐	☐
_____	☐	☐
_____	☐	☐
_____	☐	☐
_____	☐	☐
_____	☐	☐

Front   *Back*

What about your...?   Feeling sick?

Mood   ① ② ③ ④ ⑤ ⑥ ⑦ ⑧ ⑨ ⑩   ☐ Nope!

Energy levels   ① ② ③ ④ ⑤ ⑥ ⑦ ⑧ ⑨ ⑩   ☐ Yes...

Mental clarity   ① ② ③ ④ ⑤ ⑥ ⑦ ⑧ ⑨ ⑩

☐ Nausea   ☐ Diarrhea   ☐ Vomiting   ☐ Sore throat

☐ Congestion   ☐ Coughing   ☐ Chills   ☐ Fever

Other symptoms: _____

LET'S EXPLORE SOME MORE #27

Hours of Sleep ① ② ③ ④ ⑤ ⑥ ⑦ ⑧ ⑨ ⑩ ⊕

Sleep Quality ① ② ③ ④ ⑤ ⑥ ⑦ ⑧ ⑨ ⑩

WEATHER

☐ Hot ☐ Mild ☐ Cold BM Pressure: _____

☐ Dry ☐ Humid ☐ Wet Allergen Levels: _____

STRESS LEVELS

None	Low	Medium	High	Max	@$#%!

FOOD / MEDICATIONS

FOOD / DRINKS	MEDS / SUPPLEMENTS	TIME	DOSE

☐ usual daily medication

EXERCISE / DAILY ACTIVITY

☐ Damn right, I worked out.

☐ I managed to exercise a bit.

☐ No, I haven't exercised at all.

☐ I did some stuff, and that counts.

DETAILS

NOTES / TRIGGERS / IMPROVEMENTS

WRITE ONE THING YOU'RE GRATEFUL FOR

Date: _____

How are you feeling today?

Like death	Like shit	Not good	Meh	Good	Great!	Amazing!

RATE YOUR PAIN LEVEL

(1) (2) (3) (4) (5) (6) (7) (8) (9) (10)

Describe your pain / symptoms

	am	pm
	☐	☐
	☐	☐
	☐	☐
	☐	☐
	☐	☐
	☐	☐
	☐	☐
	☐	☐

Where do you feel it?

Front   *Back*

What about your...?

Mood	① ② ③ ④ ⑤ ⑥ ⑦ ⑧ ⑨ ⑩
Energy levels	① ② ③ ④ ⑤ ⑥ ⑦ ⑧ ⑨ ⑩
Mental clarity	① ② ③ ④ ⑤ ⑥ ⑦ ⑧ ⑨ ⑩

Feeling sick?

☐ Nope!

☐ Yes...

☐ Nausea ☐ Diarrhea ☐ Vomiting ☐ Sore throat

☐ Congestion ☐ Coughing ☐ Chills ☐ Fever

Other symptoms: _____

LET'S EXPLORE SOME MORE #28

Hours of Sleep ① ② ③ ④ ⑤ ⑥ ⑦ ⑧ ⑨ ⑩ ⊕

Sleep Quality ① ② ③ ④ ⑤ ⑥ ⑦ ⑧ ⑨ ⑩

WEATHER

☐ Hot ☐ Mild ☐ Cold BM Pressure: _____

☐ Dry ☐ Humid ☐ Wet Allergen Levels: _____

STRESS LEVELS

None	Low	Medium	High	Max	@$#%!

FOOD / MEDICATIONS

FOOD / DRINKS	MEDS / SUPPLEMENTS	TIME	DOSE

☐ usual daily medication

EXERCISE / DAILY ACTIVITY

DETAILS

☐ Damn right, I worked out.

☐ I managed to exercise a bit.

☐ No, I haven't exercised at all.

☐ I did some stuff, and that counts.

NOTES / TRIGGERS / IMPROVEMENTS

WRITE ONE THING YOU'RE GRATEFUL FOR

Date: _____

How are you feeling today?

Like death	Like shit	Not good	Meh	Good	Great!	Amazing!

RATE YOUR PAIN LEVEL

① ② ③ ④ ⑤ ⑥ ⑦ ⑧ ⑨ ⑩

Describe your pain / symptoms

	am	pm
	☐	☐
	☐	☐
	☐	☐
	☐	☐
	☐	☐
	☐	☐
	☐	☐
	☐	☐

Where do you feel it?

Front   *Back*

What about your...?

Mood	①	②	③	④	⑤	⑥	⑦	⑧	⑨	⑩	
Energy levels	①	②	③	④	⑤	⑥	⑦	⑧	⑨	⑩	
Mental clarity	①	②	③	④	⑤	⑥	⑦	⑧	⑨	⑩	

Feeling sick?

☐ Nope!

☐ Yes...

☐ Nausea   ☐ Diarrhea   ☐ Vomiting   ☐ Sore throat

☐ Congestion ☐ Coughing   ☐ Chills   ☐ Fever

Other symptoms:

LET'S EXPLORE SOME MORE #29

Hours of Sleep ① ② ③ ④ ⑤ ⑥ ⑦ ⑧ ⑨ ⑩ ⊕

Sleep Quality ① ② ③ ④ ⑤ ⑥ ⑦ ⑧ ⑨ ⑩

WEATHER

☐ Hot ☐ Mild ☐ Cold BM Pressure: _____

☐ Dry ☐ Humid ☐ Wet Allergen Levels: _____

STRESS LEVELS

| None | Low | Medium | High | Max | @$#%! |

FOOD / MEDICATIONS

FOOD / DRINKS	MEDS / SUPPLEMENTS	TIME	DOSE

☐ usual daily medication

EXERCISE / DAILY ACTIVITY

☐ Damn right, I worked out.

☐ I managed to exercise a bit.

☐ No, I haven't exercised at all.

☐ I did some stuff, and that counts.

DETAILS

NOTES / TRIGGERS / IMPROVEMENTS

_____

_____

_____

WRITE ONE THING YOU'RE GRATEFUL FOR

_____

Date: _____

How are you feeling today?

Like death   Like shit   Not good   Meh   Good   Great!   Amazing!

RATE YOUR PAIN LEVEL

(1) (2) (3) (4) (5) (6) (7) (8) (9) (10)

Describe your pain / symptoms			Where do you feel it?	
	am	pm	*Front*	*Back*
_____	☐	☐		
_____	☐	☐		
_____	☐	☐		
_____	☐	☐		
_____	☐	☐		
_____	☐	☐		
_____	☐	☐		
_____	☐	☐		

What about your…?   Feeling sick?

Mood	(1)(2)(3)(4)(5)(6)(7)(8)(9)(10)	☐ Nope!
Energy levels	(1)(2)(3)(4)(5)(6)(7)(8)(9)(10)	☐ Yes…
Mental clarity	(1)(2)(3)(4)(5)(6)(7)(8)(9)(10)	

☐ Nausea	☐ Diarrhea	☐ Vomiting	☐ Sore throat
☐ Congestion	☐ Coughing	☐ Chills	☐ Fever

Other symptoms: _____

LET'S EXPLORE SOME MORE #30

Hours of Sleep ① ② ③ ④ ⑤ ⑥ ⑦ ⑧ ⑨ ⑩ ⊕
Sleep Quality ① ② ③ ④ ⑤ ⑥ ⑦ ⑧ ⑨ ⑩

WEATHER

☐ Hot   ☐ Mild   ☐ Cold   BM Pressure: _____
☐ Dry   ☐ Humid   ☐ Wet   Allergen Levels: _____

STRESS LEVELS

| None | Low | Medium | High | Max | @$#%! |

FOOD / MEDICATIONS

FOOD / DRINKS	MEDS / SUPPLEMENTS	TIME	DOSE

☐ usual daily medication

EXERCISE / DAILY ACTIVITY

☐ Damn right, I worked out.
☐ I managed to exercise a bit.
☐ No, I haven't exercised at all.
☐ I did some stuff, and that counts.

DETAILS

NOTES / TRIGGERS / IMPROVEMENTS

WRITE ONE THING YOU'RE GRATEFUL FOR

Date: _____

How are you feeling today?

Like death	Like shit	Not good	Meh	Good	Great!	Amazing!

RATE YOUR PAIN LEVEL

① ② ③ ④ ⑤ ⑥ ⑦ ⑧ ⑨ ⑩

Describe your pain / symptoms

	am	pm
_____	☐	☐
_____	☐	☐
_____	☐	☐
_____	☐	☐
_____	☐	☐
_____	☐	☐
_____	☐	☐
_____	☐	☐

Where do you feel it?

Front *Back*

What about your...?

Mood	① ② ③ ④ ⑤ ⑥ ⑦ ⑧ ⑨ ⑩
Energy levels	① ② ③ ④ ⑤ ⑥ ⑦ ⑧ ⑨ ⑩
Mental clarity	① ② ③ ④ ⑤ ⑥ ⑦ ⑧ ⑨ ⑩

Feeling sick?

☐ Nope!

☐ Yes...

☐ Nausea ☐ Diarrhea ☐ Vomiting ☐ Sore throat

☐ Congestion ☐ Coughing ☐ Chills ☐ Fever

Other symptoms: _____

Hours of Sleep ① ② ③ ④ ⑤ ⑥ ⑦ ⑧ ⑨ ⑩ ⊕
Sleep Quality ① ② ③ ④ ⑤ ⑥ ⑦ ⑧ ⑨ ⑩

WEATHER

☐ Hot ☐ Mild ☐ Cold BM Pressure: _____
☐ Dry ☐ Humid ☐ Wet Allergen Levels: _____

STRESS LEVELS

None	Low	Medium	High	Max	@$#%!

FOOD / MEDICATIONS

FOOD / DRINKS	MEDS / SUPPLEMENTS	TIME	DOSE

☐ usual daily medication

EXERCISE / DAILY ACTIVITY

☐ Damn right, I worked out.
☐ I managed to exercise a bit.
☐ No, I haven't exercised at all.
☐ I did some stuff, and that counts.

DETAILS

NOTES / TRIGGERS / IMPROVEMENTS

WRITE ONE THING YOU'RE GRATEFUL FOR

Date: _____

How are you feeling today?

Like death	Like shit	Not good	Meh	Good	Great!	Amazing!

RATE YOUR PAIN LEVEL

(1) (2) (3) (4) (5) (6) (7) (8) (9) (10)

Describe your pain / symptoms

	am	pm
	☐	☐
	☐	☐
	☐	☐
	☐	☐
	☐	☐
	☐	☐
	☐	☐
	☐	☐

Where do you feel it?

Front   *Back*

What about your...?

Mood	(1)(2)(3)(4)(5)(6)(7)(8)(9)(10)
Energy levels	(1)(2)(3)(4)(5)(6)(7)(8)(9)(10)
Mental clarity	(1)(2)(3)(4)(5)(6)(7)(8)(9)(10)

Feeling sick?

☐ Nope!

☐ Yes...

☐ Nausea   ☐ Diarrhea   ☐ Vomiting   ☐ Sore throat

☐ Congestion ☐ Coughing   ☐ Chills   ☐ Fever

Other symptoms: _____

LET'S EXPLORE SOME MORE #32

Hours of Sleep (1) (2) (3) (4) (5) (6) (7) (8) (9) (10) (+)

Sleep Quality (1) (2) (3) (4) (5) (6) (7) (8) (9) (10)

WEATHER

☐ Hot   ☐ Mild   ☐ Cold   BM Pressure: _____

☐ Dry   ☐ Humid   ☐ Wet   Allergen Levels: _____

STRESS LEVELS

None	Low	Medium	High	Max	@$#%!

FOOD / MEDICATIONS

FOOD / DRINKS	MEDS / SUPPLEMENTS	TIME	DOSE

☐ usual daily medication

EXERCISE / DAILY ACTIVITY

☐ Damn right, I worked out.

☐ I managed to exercise a bit.

☐ No, I haven't exercised at all.

☐ I did some stuff, and that counts.

DETAILS

NOTES / TRIGGERS / IMPROVEMENTS

WRITE ONE THING YOU'RE GRATEFUL FOR

Date: _____

How are you feeling today?

Like death	Like shit	Not good	Meh	Good	Great!	Amazing!

RATE YOUR PAIN LEVEL

① ② ③ ④ ⑤ ⑥ ⑦ ⑧ ⑨ ⑩

Describe your pain / symptoms

	am	pm
_____	☐	☐
_____	☐	☐
_____	☐	☐
_____	☐	☐
_____	☐	☐
_____	☐	☐
_____	☐	☐
_____	☐	☐

Where do you feel it?

Front   *Back*

What about your...?

Mood	① ② ③ ④ ⑤ ⑥ ⑦ ⑧ ⑨ ⑩
Energy levels	① ② ③ ④ ⑤ ⑥ ⑦ ⑧ ⑨ ⑩
Mental clarity	① ② ③ ④ ⑤ ⑥ ⑦ ⑧ ⑨ ⑩

Feeling sick?

☐ Nope!

☐ Yes...

☐ Nausea   ☐ Diarrhea   ☐ Vomiting   ☐ Sore throat

☐ Congestion   ☐ Coughing   ☐ Chills   ☐ Fever

Other symptoms: _____

LET'S EXPLORE SOME MORE #33

Hours of Sleep ① ② ③ ④ ⑤ ⑥ ⑦ ⑧ ⑨ ⑩ ⊕
Sleep Quality ① ② ③ ④ ⑤ ⑥ ⑦ ⑧ ⑨ ⑩

WEATHER

☐ Hot   ☐ Mild   ☐ Cold   BM Pressure: _____

☐ Dry   ☐ Humid ☐ Wet   Allergen Levels: _____

STRESS LEVELS

None	Low	Medium	High	Max	@$#%!

FOOD / MEDICATIONS

FOOD / DRINKS	MEDS / SUPPLEMENTS	TIME	DOSE

☐ usual daily medication

EXERCISE / DAILY ACTIVITY

☐ Damn right, I worked out.

☐ I managed to exercise a bit.

☐ No, I haven't exercised at all.

☐ I did some stuff, and that counts.

DETAILS

NOTES / TRIGGERS / IMPROVEMENTS

WRITE ONE THING YOU'RE GRATEFUL FOR

Date: _____

How are you feeling today?

| Like death | Like shit | Not good | Meh | Good | Great! | Amazing! |

RATE YOUR PAIN LEVEL

(1) (2) (3) (4) (5) (6) (7) (8) (9) (10)

Describe your pain / symptoms

	am	pm
_____	☐	☐
_____	☐	☐
_____	☐	☐
_____	☐	☐
_____	☐	☐
_____	☐	☐
_____	☐	☐
_____	☐	☐

Where do you feel it?

Front   *Back*

What about your...?

Mood	(1) (2) (3) (4) (5) (6) (7) (8) (9) (10)
Energy levels	(1) (2) (3) (4) (5) (6) (7) (8) (9) (10)
Mental clarity	(1) (2) (3) (4) (5) (6) (7) (8) (9) (10)

Feeling sick?

☐ Nope!

☐ Yes...

☐ Nausea   ☐ Diarrhea   ☐ Vomiting   ☐ Sore throat

☐ Congestion   ☐ Coughing   ☐ Chills   ☐ Fever

Other symptoms: _____

LET'S EXPLORE SOME MORE #34

Hours of Sleep ① ② ③ ④ ⑤ ⑥ ⑦ ⑧ ⑨ ⑩ ⊕
Sleep Quality ① ② ③ ④ ⑤ ⑥ ⑦ ⑧ ⑨ ⑩

WEATHER

☐ Hot   ☐ Mild   ☐ Cold   BM Pressure: _____
☐ Dry   ☐ Humid   ☐ Wet   Allergen Levels: _____

STRESS LEVELS

None	Low	Medium	High	Max	@$#%!

FOOD / MEDICATIONS

FOOD / DRINKS	MEDS / SUPPLEMENTS	TIME	DOSE

☐ usual daily medication

EXERCISE / DAILY ACTIVITY

☐ Damn right, I worked out.
☐ I managed to exercise a bit.
☐ No, I haven't exercised at all.
☐ I did some stuff, and that counts.

DETAILS

NOTES / TRIGGERS / IMPROVEMENTS

_____
_____
_____

WRITE ONE THING YOU'RE GRATEFUL FOR
_____

Date: _____

How are you feeling today?

Like death	Like shit	Not good	Meh	Good	Great!	Amazing!

RATE YOUR PAIN LEVEL

(1) (2) (3) (4) (5) (6) (7) (8) (9) (10)

Describe your pain / symptoms

	am	pm
	☐	☐
	☐	☐
	☐	☐
	☐	☐
	☐	☐
	☐	☐
	☐	☐
	☐	☐

Where do you feel it?

Front   *Back*

What about your...?

Mood	(1) (2) (3) (4) (5) (6) (7) (8) (9) (10)
Energy levels	(1) (2) (3) (4) (5) (6) (7) (8) (9) (10)
Mental clarity	(1) (2) (3) (4) (5) (6) (7) (8) (9) (10)

Feeling sick?

☐ Nope!

☐ Yes...

☐ Nausea   ☐ Diarrhea   ☐ Vomiting   ☐ Sore throat

☐ Congestion   ☐ Coughing   ☐ Chills   ☐ Fever

Other symptoms:

LET'S EXPLORE SOME MORE #35

Hours of Sleep ① ② ③ ④ ⑤ ⑥ ⑦ ⑧ ⑨ ⑩ ⊕

Sleep Quality ① ② ③ ④ ⑤ ⑥ ⑦ ⑧ ⑨ ⑩

WEATHER

☐ Hot   ☐ Mild   ☐ Cold   BM Pressure: _____

☐ Dry   ☐ Humid   ☐ Wet   Allergen Levels: _____

STRESS LEVELS

None	Low	Medium	High	Max	@$#%!

FOOD / MEDICATIONS

FOOD / DRINKS	MEDS / SUPPLEMENTS	TIME	DOSE

☐ usual daily medication

EXERCISE / DAILY ACTIVITY

☐ Damn right, I worked out.

☐ I managed to exercise a bit.

☐ No, I haven't exercised at all.

☐ I did some stuff, and that counts.

DETAILS

NOTES / TRIGGERS / IMPROVEMENTS

_____

_____

_____

WRITE ONE THING YOU'RE GRATEFUL FOR

_____

Date: _____

How are you feeling today?

Like death | Like shit | Not good | Meh | Good | Great! | Amazing!

RATE YOUR PAIN LEVEL

① ② ③ ④ ⑤ ⑥ ⑦ ⑧ ⑨ ⑩

Describe your pain / symptoms

	am	pm
_____	☐	☐
_____	☐	☐
_____	☐	☐
_____	☐	☐
_____	☐	☐
_____	☐	☐
_____	☐	☐
_____	☐	☐

Where do you feel it?

Front   *Back*

What about your...?

Mood   ① ② ③ ④ ⑤ ⑥ ⑦ ⑧ ⑨ ⑩
Energy levels   ① ② ③ ④ ⑤ ⑥ ⑦ ⑧ ⑨ ⑩
Mental clarity   ① ② ③ ④ ⑤ ⑥ ⑦ ⑧ ⑨ ⑩

Feeling sick?

☐ Nope!
☐ Yes...

☐ Nausea   ☐ Diarrhea   ☐ Vomiting   ☐ Sore throat
☐ Congestion   ☐ Coughing   ☐ Chills   ☐ Fever

Other symptoms: _____

Hours of Sleep (1)(2)(3)(4)(5)(6)(7)(8)(9)(10)(+)

Sleep Quality (1)(2)(3)(4)(5)(6)(7)(8)(9)(10)

WEATHER

☐ Hot   ☐ Mild   ☐ Cold   BM Pressure: _____

☐ Dry   ☐ Humid ☐ Wet   Allergen Levels: _____

STRESS LEVELS

None	Low	Medium	High	Max	@$#%!

FOOD / MEDICATIONS

FOOD / DRINKS	MEDS / SUPPLEMENTS	TIME	DOSE

☐ usual daily medication

EXERCISE / DAILY ACTIVITY

☐ Damn right, I worked out.

☐ I managed to exercise a bit.

☐ No, I haven't exercised at all.

☐ I did some stuff, and that counts.

DETAILS

NOTES / TRIGGERS / IMPROVEMENTS

WRITE ONE THING YOU'RE GRATEFUL FOR

Date: _____

How are you feeling today?

| Like death | Like shit | Not good | Meh | Good | Great! | Amazing! |

RATE YOUR PAIN LEVEL

① ② ③ ④ ⑤ ⑥ ⑦ ⑧ ⑨ ⑩

Describe your pain / symptoms

	am	pm
_____	☐	☐
_____	☐	☐
_____	☐	☐
_____	☐	☐
_____	☐	☐
_____	☐	☐
_____	☐	☐
_____	☐	☐

Where do you feel it?

Front   *Back*

What about your...?

Mood	① ② ③ ④ ⑤ ⑥ ⑦ ⑧ ⑨ ⑩
Energy levels	① ② ③ ④ ⑤ ⑥ ⑦ ⑧ ⑨ ⑩
Mental clarity	① ② ③ ④ ⑤ ⑥ ⑦ ⑧ ⑨ ⑩

Feeling sick?

☐ Nope!

☐ Yes...

☐ Nausea   ☐ Diarrhea   ☐ Vomiting   ☐ Sore throat

☐ Congestion ☐ Coughing   ☐ Chills   ☐ Fever

Other symptoms: _____

LET'S EXPLORE SOME MORE #37

Hours of Sleep (1) (2) (3) (4) (5) (6) (7) (8) (9) (10) (+)
Sleep Quality (1) (2) (3) (4) (5) (6) (7) (8) (9) (10)

WEATHER

☐ Hot ☐ Mild ☐ Cold BM Pressure: _____

☐ Dry ☐ Humid ☐ Wet Allergen Levels: _____

STRESS LEVELS

None	Low	Medium	High	Max	@$#%!

FOOD / MEDICATIONS

FOOD / DRINKS	MEDS / SUPPLEMENTS	TIME	DOSE

☐ usual daily medication

EXERCISE / DAILY ACTIVITY

DETAILS

☐ Damn right, I worked out.

☐ I managed to exercise a bit.

☐ No, I haven't exercised at all.

☐ I did some stuff, and that counts.

NOTES / TRIGGERS / IMPROVEMENTS

_____

_____

_____

WRITE ONE THING YOU'RE GRATEFUL FOR

_____

Date: _____

How are you feeling today?

Like death	Like shit	Not good	Meh	Good	Great!	Amazing!

RATE YOUR PAIN LEVEL

① ② ③ ④ ⑤ ⑥ ⑦ ⑧ ⑨ ⑩

Describe your pain / symptoms

	am	pm
	☐	☐
	☐	☐
	☐	☐
	☐	☐
	☐	☐
	☐	☐
	☐	☐
	☐	☐

Where do you feel it?

Front   Back

What about your...?

Mood	① ② ③ ④ ⑤ ⑥ ⑦ ⑧ ⑨ ⑩
Energy levels	① ② ③ ④ ⑤ ⑥ ⑦ ⑧ ⑨ ⑩
Mental clarity	① ② ③ ④ ⑤ ⑥ ⑦ ⑧ ⑨ ⑩

Feeling sick?

☐ Nope!
☐ Yes...

☐ Nausea   ☐ Diarrhea   ☐ Vomiting   ☐ Sore throat
☐ Congestion   ☐ Coughing   ☐ Chills   ☐ Fever

Other symptoms: _____

LET'S EXPLORE SOME MORE #38

Hours of Sleep ① ② ③ ④ ⑤ ⑥ ⑦ ⑧ ⑨ ⑩ ⊕
Sleep Quality ① ② ③ ④ ⑤ ⑥ ⑦ ⑧ ⑨ ⑩

WEATHER

☐ Hot ☐ Mild ☐ Cold BM Pressure: _____

☐ Dry ☐ Humid ☐ Wet Allergen Levels: _____

STRESS LEVELS

None	Low	Medium	High	Max	@$#%!

FOOD / MEDICATIONS

FOOD / DRINKS	MEDS / SUPPLEMENTS	TIME	DOSE

☐ usual daily medication

EXERCISE / DAILY ACTIVITY

☐ Damn right, I worked out.

☐ I managed to exercise a bit.

☐ No, I haven't exercised at all.

☐ I did some stuff, and that counts.

DETAILS

NOTES / TRIGGERS / IMPROVEMENTS

_____

_____

_____

WRITE ONE THING YOU'RE GRATEFUL FOR

_____

Date: _____

How are you feeling today?

Like death	Like shit	Not good	Meh	Good	Great!	Amazing!

RATE YOUR PAIN LEVEL

① ② ③ ④ ⑤ ⑥ ⑦ ⑧ ⑨ ⑩

Describe your pain / symptoms   Where do you feel it?

	am	pm
_____	☐	☐
_____	☐	☐
_____	☐	☐
_____	☐	☐
_____	☐	☐
_____	☐	☐
_____	☐	☐
	☐	☐

Front   *Back*

What about your...?   Feeling sick?

Mood ① ② ③ ④ ⑤ ⑥ ⑦ ⑧ ⑨ ⑩   ☐ Nope!

Energy levels ① ② ③ ④ ⑤ ⑥ ⑦ ⑧ ⑨ ⑩   ☐ Yes...

Mental clarity ① ② ③ ④ ⑤ ⑥ ⑦ ⑧ ⑨ ⑩

☐ Nausea   ☐ Diarrhea   ☐ Vomiting   ☐ Sore throat

☐ Congestion   ☐ Coughing   ☐ Chills   ☐ Fever

Other symptoms: _____

LET'S EXPLORE SOME MORE #39

Hours of Sleep ① ② ③ ④ ⑤ ⑥ ⑦ ⑧ ⑨ ⑩ ⊕

Sleep Quality ① ② ③ ④ ⑤ ⑥ ⑦ ⑧ ⑨ ⑩

WEATHER

☐ Hot   ☐ Mild   ☐ Cold   BM Pressure: _____

☐ Dry   ☐ Humid   ☐ Wet   Allergen Levels: _____

STRESS LEVELS

| None | Low | Medium | High | Max | @$#%! |

FOOD / MEDICATIONS

FOOD / DRINKS	MEDS / SUPPLEMENTS	TIME	DOSE
	☐ usual daily medication		

EXERCISE / DAILY ACTIVITY

☐ Damn right, I worked out.

☐ I managed to exercise a bit.

☐ No, I haven't exercised at all.

☐ I did some stuff, and that counts.

DETAILS

NOTES / TRIGGERS / IMPROVEMENTS

WRITE ONE THING YOU'RE GRATEFUL FOR

Date: _____

How are you feeling today?

Like death	Like shit	Not good	Meh	Good	Great!	Amazing!

RATE YOUR PAIN LEVEL

(1) (2) (3) (4) (5) (6) (7) (8) (9) (10)

Describe your pain / symptoms

	am	pm
_____	☐	☐
_____	☐	☐
_____	☐	☐
_____	☐	☐
_____	☐	☐
_____	☐	☐
_____	☐	☐
_____	☐	☐

Where do you feel it?

Front   *Back*

What about your...?

Mood	(1) (2) (3) (4) (5) (6) (7) (8) (9) (10)
Energy levels	(1) (2) (3) (4) (5) (6) (7) (8) (9) (10)
Mental clarity	(1) (2) (3) (4) (5) (6) (7) (8) (9) (10)

Feeling sick?

☐ Nope!

☐ Yes...

☐ Nausea   ☐ Diarrhea   ☐ Vomiting   ☐ Sore throat

☐ Congestion   ☐ Coughing   ☐ Chills   ☐ Fever

Other symptoms: _____

LET'S EXPLORE SOME MORE #40

Hours of Sleep (1) (2) (3) (4) (5) (6) (7) (8) (9) (10) (+)

Sleep Quality (1) (2) (3) (4) (5) (6) (7) (8) (9) (10)

WEATHER

☐ Hot   ☐ Mild   ☐ Cold   BM Pressure: _____

☐ Dry   ☐ Humid   ☐ Wet   Allergen Levels: _____

STRESS LEVELS

| None | Low | Medium | High | Max | @$#%! |

FOOD / MEDICATIONS

FOOD / DRINKS	MEDS / SUPPLEMENTS	TIME	DOSE
	☐ usual daily medication		

EXERCISE / DAILY ACTIVITY

DETAILS

☐ Damn right, I worked out.

☐ I managed to exercise a bit.

☐ No, I haven't exercised at all.

☐ I did some stuff, and that counts.

NOTES / TRIGGERS / IMPROVEMENTS

_____

_____

_____

WRITE ONE THING YOU'RE GRATEFUL FOR

_____

How are you feeling today?

Like death	Like shit	Not good	Meh	Good	Great!	Amazing!

RATE YOUR PAIN LEVEL

① ② ③ ④ ⑤ ⑥ ⑦ ⑧ ⑨ ⑩

Describe your pain / symptoms

	am	pm
	☐	☐
	☐	☐
	☐	☐
	☐	☐
	☐	☐
	☐	☐
	☐	☐
	☐	☐

Where do you feel it?

Front　　*Back*

What about your...?

Mood ① ② ③ ④ ⑤ ⑥ ⑦ ⑧ ⑨ ⑩

Energy levels ① ② ③ ④ ⑤ ⑥ ⑦ ⑧ ⑨ ⑩

Mental clarity ① ② ③ ④ ⑤ ⑥ ⑦ ⑧ ⑨ ⑩

Feeling sick?

☐ Nope!

☐ Yes...

☐ Nausea ☐ Diarrhea ☐ Vomiting ☐ Sore throat

☐ Congestion ☐ Coughing ☐ Chills ☐ Fever

Other symptoms: _____

LET'S EXPLORE SOME MORE #41

Hours of Sleep ① ② ③ ④ ⑤ ⑥ ⑦ ⑧ ⑨ ⑩ ⊕

Sleep Quality ① ② ③ ④ ⑤ ⑥ ⑦ ⑧ ⑨ ⑩

WEATHER

☐ Hot   ☐ Mild   ☐ Cold   BM Pressure: _____

☐ Dry   ☐ Humid   ☐ Wet   Allergen Levels: _____

STRESS LEVELS

None	Low	Medium	High	Max	@$#%!

FOOD / MEDICATIONS

FOOD / DRINKS	MEDS / SUPPLEMENTS	TIME	DOSE

☐ usual daily medication

EXERCISE / DAILY ACTIVITY

☐ Damn right, I worked out.

☐ I managed to exercise a bit.

☐ No, I haven't exercised at all.

☐ I did some stuff, and that counts.

DETAILS

NOTES / TRIGGERS / IMPROVEMENTS

_____

_____

_____

WRITE ONE THING YOU'RE GRATEFUL FOR

_____

Date: _____

How are you feeling today?

x x	>;<	☹	☺	☺	😁	😍
Like death	Like shit	Not good	Meh	Good	Great!	Amazing!

RATE YOUR PAIN LEVEL

① ② ③ ④ ⑤ ⑥ ⑦ ⑧ ⑨ ⑩

Describe your pain / symptoms   Where do you feel it?

	am	pm
	☐	☐
	☐	☐
	☐	☐
	☐	☐
	☐	☐
	☐	☐
	☐	☐
	☐	☐

Front   *Back*

What about your...?   Feeling sick?

Mood   ① ② ③ ④ ⑤ ⑥ ⑦ ⑧ ⑨ ⑩   ☐ Nope!
Energy levels ① ② ③ ④ ⑤ ⑥ ⑦ ⑧ ⑨ ⑩   ☐ Yes...
Mental clarity ① ② ③ ④ ⑤ ⑥ ⑦ ⑧ ⑨ ⑩

☐ Nausea   ☐ Diarrhea   ☐ Vomiting   ☐ Sore throat
☐ Congestion ☐ Coughing   ☐ Chills   ☐ Fever

Other symptoms: _____

LET'S EXPLORE SOME MORE

Hours of Sleep (1)(2)(3)(4)(5)(6)(7)(8)(9)(10)(+)

Sleep Quality (1)(2)(3)(4)(5)(6)(7)(8)(9)(10)

WEATHER

☐ Hot ☐ Mild ☐ Cold BM Pressure: _____

☐ Dry ☐ Humid ☐ Wet Allergen Levels: _____

STRESS LEVELS

None	Low	Medium	High	Max	@$#%!

FOOD / MEDICATIONS

FOOD / DRINKS	MEDS / SUPPLEMENTS	TIME	DOSE

☐ usual daily medication

EXERCISE / DAILY ACTIVITY

DETAILS

☐ Damn right, I worked out.

☐ I managed to exercise a bit.

☐ No, I haven't exercised at all.

☐ I did some stuff, and that counts.

NOTES / TRIGGERS / IMPROVEMENTS

_____

_____

_____

WRITE ONE THING YOU'RE GRATEFUL FOR

_____

Date: _____

How are you feeling today?

| Like death | Like shit | Not good | Meh | Good | Great! | Amazing! |

RATE YOUR PAIN LEVEL

① ② ③ ④ ⑤ ⑥ ⑦ ⑧ ⑨ ⑩

Describe your pain / symptoms

Where do you feel it?

	am	pm
_____	☐	☐
_____	☐	☐
_____	☐	☐
_____	☐	☐
_____	☐	☐
_____	☐	☐
_____	☐	☐
_____	☐	☐

Front　　*Back*

What about your...?

Feeling sick?

Mood	① ② ③ ④ ⑤ ⑥ ⑦ ⑧ ⑨ ⑩	☐ Nope!
Energy levels	① ② ③ ④ ⑤ ⑥ ⑦ ⑧ ⑨ ⑩	☐ Yes...
Mental clarity	① ② ③ ④ ⑤ ⑥ ⑦ ⑧ ⑨ ⑩	

☐ Nausea　　☐ Diarrhea　　☐ Vomiting　　☐ Sore throat

☐ Congestion　　☐ Coughing　　☐ Chills　　☐ Fever

Other symptoms: _____

LET'S EXPLORE SOME MORE #43

Hours of Sleep ① ② ③ ④ ⑤ ⑥ ⑦ ⑧ ⑨ ⑩ ⊕

Sleep Quality ① ② ③ ④ ⑤ ⑥ ⑦ ⑧ ⑨ ⑩

WEATHER

☐ Hot ☐ Mild ☐ Cold BM Pressure: _____

☐ Dry ☐ Humid ☐ Wet Allergen Levels: _____

STRESS LEVELS

None	Low	Medium	High	Max	@$#%!

FOOD / MEDICATIONS

FOOD / DRINKS	MEDS / SUPPLEMENTS	TIME	DOSE

☐ usual daily medication

EXERCISE / DAILY ACTIVITY

☐ Damn right, I worked out.

☐ I managed to exercise a bit.

☐ No, I haven't exercised at all.

☐ I did some stuff, and that counts.

DETAILS

NOTES / TRIGGERS / IMPROVEMENTS

WRITE ONE THING YOU'RE GRATEFUL FOR

Date: _____

How are you feeling today?

| Like death | Like shit | Not good | Meh | Good | Great! | Amazing! |

RATE YOUR PAIN LEVEL

(1) (2) (3) (4) (5) (6) (7) (8) (9) (10)

Describe your pain / symptoms

	am	pm
_____	☐	☐
_____	☐	☐
_____	☐	☐
_____	☐	☐
_____	☐	☐
_____	☐	☐
_____	☐	☐
_____	☐	☐

Where do you feel it?

Front   *Back*

What about your...?

Mood	(1) (2) (3) (4) (5) (6) (7) (8) (9) (10)
Energy levels	(1) (2) (3) (4) (5) (6) (7) (8) (9) (10)
Mental clarity	(1) (2) (3) (4) (5) (6) (7) (8) (9) (10)

Feeling sick?

☐ Nope!

☐ Yes...

☐ Nausea ☐ Diarrhea ☐ Vomiting ☐ Sore throat

☐ Congestion ☐ Coughing ☐ Chills ☐ Fever

Other symptoms: _____

LET'S EXPLORE SOME MORE #44

Hours of Sleep ① ② ③ ④ ⑤ ⑥ ⑦ ⑧ ⑨ ⑩ ⊕
Sleep Quality ① ② ③ ④ ⑤ ⑥ ⑦ ⑧ ⑨ ⑩

WEATHER

☐ Hot   ☐ Mild   ☐ Cold   BM Pressure: _____

☐ Dry   ☐ Humid   ☐ Wet   Allergen Levels: _____

STRESS LEVELS

None	Low	Medium	High	Max	@$#%!

FOOD / MEDICATIONS

FOOD / DRINKS	MEDS / SUPPLEMENTS	TIME	DOSE

☐ usual daily medication

EXERCISE / DAILY ACTIVITY

☐ Damn right, I worked out.

☐ I managed to exercise a bit.

☐ No, I haven't exercised at all.

☐ I did some stuff, and that counts.

DETAILS

NOTES / TRIGGERS / IMPROVEMENTS

_____

_____

_____

WRITE ONE THING YOU'RE GRATEFUL FOR

_____

Date: _____

How are you feeling today?

Like death   Like shit   Not good   Meh   Good   Great!   Amazing!

RATE YOUR PAIN LEVEL

(1) (2) (3) (4) (5) (6) (7) (8) (9) (10)

Describe your pain / symptoms			Where do you feel it?

Describe your pain / symptoms

	am	pm
	☐	☐
	☐	☐
	☐	☐
	☐	☐
	☐	☐
	☐	☐
	☐	☐
	☐	☐

Where do you feel it?

Front   *Back*

What about your...?

		Feeling sick?
Mood	(1)(2)(3)(4)(5)(6)(7)(8)(9)(10)	☐ Nope!
Energy levels	(1)(2)(3)(4)(5)(6)(7)(8)(9)(10)	☐ Yes...
Mental clarity	(1)(2)(3)(4)(5)(6)(7)(8)(9)(10)	

☐ Nausea   ☐ Diarrhea   ☐ Vomiting   ☐ Sore throat

☐ Congestion   ☐ Coughing   ☐ Chills   ☐ Fever

Other symptoms: _____

Hours of Sleep ① ② ③ ④ ⑤ ⑥ ⑦ ⑧ ⑨ ⑩ ⊕
Sleep Quality ① ② ③ ④ ⑤ ⑥ ⑦ ⑧ ⑨ ⑩

WEATHER

☐ Hot   ☐ Mild   ☐ Cold   BM Pressure: _____

☐ Dry   ☐ Humid   ☐ Wet   Allergen Levels: _____

STRESS LEVELS

None	Low	Medium	High	Max	@$#%!

FOOD / MEDICATIONS

FOOD / DRINKS	MEDS / SUPPLEMENTS	TIME	DOSE

☐ usual daily medication

EXERCISE / DAILY ACTIVITY

☐ Damn right, I worked out.

☐ I managed to exercise a bit.

☐ No, I haven't exercised at all.

☐ I did some stuff, and that counts.

DETAILS

NOTES / TRIGGERS / IMPROVEMENTS

WRITE ONE THING YOU'RE GRATEFUL FOR

Date: _____

How are you feeling today?

Like death	Like shit	Not good	Meh	Good	Great!	Amazing!

RATE YOUR PAIN LEVEL

① ② ③ ④ ⑤ ⑥ ⑦ ⑧ ⑨ ⑩

Describe your pain / symptoms

	am	pm
_____	☐	☐
_____	☐	☐
_____	☐	☐
_____	☐	☐
_____	☐	☐
_____	☐	☐
_____	☐	☐
_____	☐	☐

Where do you feel it?

Front   *Back*

What about your...?

Mood	① ② ③ ④ ⑤ ⑥ ⑦ ⑧ ⑨ ⑩
Energy levels	① ② ③ ④ ⑤ ⑥ ⑦ ⑧ ⑨ ⑩
Mental clarity	① ② ③ ④ ⑤ ⑥ ⑦ ⑧ ⑨ ⑩

Feeling sick?

☐ Nope!

☐ Yes...

☐ Nausea   ☐ Diarrhea   ☐ Vomiting   ☐ Sore throat

☐ Congestion   ☐ Coughing   ☐ Chills   ☐ Fever

Other symptoms: _____

LET'S EXPLORE SOME MORE #46

Hours of Sleep ① ② ③ ④ ⑤ ⑥ ⑦ ⑧ ⑨ ⑩ ⊕
Sleep Quality ① ② ③ ④ ⑤ ⑥ ⑦ ⑧ ⑨ ⑩

WEATHER

☐ Hot   ☐ Mild   ☐ Cold   BM Pressure: _____

☐ Dry   ☐ Humid   ☐ Wet   Allergen Levels: _____

STRESS LEVELS

None	Low	Medium	High	Max	@$#%!

FOOD / MEDICATIONS

FOOD / DRINKS	MEDS / SUPPLEMENTS	TIME	DOSE

☐ usual daily medication

EXERCISE / DAILY ACTIVITY

☐ Damn right, I worked out.

☐ I managed to exercise a bit.

☐ No, I haven't exercised at all.

☐ I did some stuff, and that counts.

DETAILS

NOTES / TRIGGERS / IMPROVEMENTS

WRITE ONE THING YOU'RE GRATEFUL FOR

Date: _____

How are you feeling today?

| Like death | Like shit | Not good | Meh | Good | Great! | Amazing! |

RATE YOUR PAIN LEVEL

① ② ③ ④ ⑤ ⑥ ⑦ ⑧ ⑨ ⑩

Describe your pain / symptoms

	am	pm
_____	☐	☐
_____	☐	☐
_____	☐	☐
_____	☐	☐
_____	☐	☐
_____	☐	☐
_____	☐	☐
_____	☐	☐

Where do you feel it?

Front   *Back*

What about your...?

Mood	① ② ③ ④ ⑤ ⑥ ⑦ ⑧ ⑨ ⑩
Energy levels	① ② ③ ④ ⑤ ⑥ ⑦ ⑧ ⑨ ⑩
Mental clarity	① ② ③ ④ ⑤ ⑥ ⑦ ⑧ ⑨ ⑩

Feeling sick?

☐ Nope!

☐ Yes...

☐ Nausea ☐ Diarrhea ☐ Vomiting ☐ Sore throat

☐ Congestion ☐ Coughing ☐ Chills ☐ Fever

Other symptoms: _____

LET'S EXPLORE SOME MORE #47

Hours of Sleep (1) (2) (3) (4) (5) (6) (7) (8) (9) (10) (+)

Sleep Quality (1) (2) (3) (4) (5) (6) (7) (8) (9) (10)

WEATHER

☐ Hot ☐ Mild ☐ Cold BM Pressure: _____

☐ Dry ☐ Humid ☐ Wet Allergen Levels: _____

STRESS LEVELS

None	Low	Medium	High	Max	@$#%!

FOOD / MEDICATIONS

FOOD / DRINKS	MEDS / SUPPLEMENTS	TIME	DOSE

☐ usual daily medication

EXERCISE / DAILY ACTIVITY

☐ Damn right, I worked out.

☐ I managed to exercise a bit.

☐ No, I haven't exercised at all.

☐ I did some stuff, and that counts.

DETAILS

NOTES / TRIGGERS / IMPROVEMENTS

WRITE ONE THING YOU'RE GRATEFUL FOR

Date: _____

How are you feeling today?

Like death	Like shit	Not good	Meh	Good	Great!	Amazing!

RATE YOUR PAIN LEVEL

① ② ③ ④ ⑤ ⑥ ⑦ ⑧ ⑨ ⑩

Describe your pain / symptoms

	am	pm
	☐	☐
	☐	☐
	☐	☐
	☐	☐
	☐	☐
	☐	☐
	☐	☐
	☐	☐

Where do you feel it?

Front   *Back*

What about your...?

Mood	① ② ③ ④ ⑤ ⑥ ⑦ ⑧ ⑨ ⑩
Energy levels	① ② ③ ④ ⑤ ⑥ ⑦ ⑧ ⑨ ⑩
Mental clarity	① ② ③ ④ ⑤ ⑥ ⑦ ⑧ ⑨ ⑩

Feeling sick?

☐ Nope!

☐ Yes...

☐ Nausea   ☐ Diarrhea   ☐ Vomiting   ☐ Sore throat

☐ Congestion   ☐ Coughing   ☐ Chills   ☐ Fever

Other symptoms: _____

LET'S EXPLORE SOME MORE #48

Hours of Sleep (1) (2) (3) (4) (5) (6) (7) (8) (9) (10) (+)

Sleep Quality (1) (2) (3) (4) (5) (6) (7) (8) (9) (10)

WEATHER

☐ Hot   ☐ Mild   ☐ Cold   BM Pressure: _____

☐ Dry   ☐ Humid   ☐ Wet   Allergen Levels: _____

STRESS LEVELS

None	Low	Medium	High	Max	@$#%!

FOOD / MEDICATIONS

FOOD / DRINKS	MEDS / SUPPLEMENTS	TIME	DOSE
	☐ usual daily medication		

EXERCISE / DAILY ACTIVITY

DETAILS

☐ Damn right, I worked out.

☐ I managed to exercise a bit.

☐ No, I haven't exercised at all.

☐ I did some stuff, and that counts.

NOTES / TRIGGERS / IMPROVEMENTS

_____

_____

_____

_____

WRITE ONE THING YOU'RE GRATEFUL FOR

_____

Date: _____

How are you feeling today?

Like death	Like shit	Not good	Meh	Good	Great!	Amazing!

RATE YOUR PAIN LEVEL

① ② ③ ④ ⑤ ⑥ ⑦ ⑧ ⑨ ⑩

Describe your pain / symptoms

	am	pm
_____	☐	☐
_____	☐	☐
_____	☐	☐
_____	☐	☐
_____	☐	☐
_____	☐	☐
_____	☐	☐
_____	☐	☐

Where do you feel it?

Front   *Back*

What about your...?

Mood	① ② ③ ④ ⑤ ⑥ ⑦ ⑧ ⑨ ⑩
Energy levels	① ② ③ ④ ⑤ ⑥ ⑦ ⑧ ⑨ ⑩
Mental clarity	① ② ③ ④ ⑤ ⑥ ⑦ ⑧ ⑨ ⑩

Feeling sick?

☐ Nope!

☐ Yes...

☐ Nausea   ☐ Diarrhea   ☐ Vomiting   ☐ Sore throat

☐ Congestion   ☐ Coughing   ☐ Chills   ☐ Fever

Other symptoms: _____

LET'S EXPLORE SOME MORE #49

Hours of Sleep ① ② ③ ④ ⑤ ⑥ ⑦ ⑧ ⑨ ⑩ ⊕
Sleep Quality ① ② ③ ④ ⑤ ⑥ ⑦ ⑧ ⑨ ⑩

WEATHER

☐ Hot ☐ Mild ☐ Cold BM Pressure: _____
☐ Dry ☐ Humid ☐ Wet Allergen Levels: _____

STRESS LEVELS

None	Low	Medium	High	Max	@$#%!

FOOD / MEDICATIONS

FOOD / DRINKS	MEDS / SUPPLEMENTS	TIME	DOSE

☐ usual daily medication

EXERCISE / DAILY ACTIVITY

☐ Damn right, I worked out.
☐ I managed to exercise a bit.
☐ No, I haven't exercised at all.
☐ I did some stuff, and that counts.

DETAILS

NOTES / TRIGGERS / IMPROVEMENTS

_____

_____

_____

WRITE ONE THING YOU'RE GRATEFUL FOR

_____

How are you feeling today?

Like death	Like shit	Not good	Meh	Good	Great!	Amazing!

RATE YOUR PAIN LEVEL

(1) (2) (3) (4) (5) (6) (7) (8) (9) (10)

Describe your pain / symptoms

	am	pm
_____	☐	☐
_____	☐	☐
_____	☐	☐
_____	☐	☐
_____	☐	☐
_____	☐	☐
_____	☐	☐
_____	☐	☐

Where do you feel it?

Front   *Back*

What about your...?

Mood	(1) (2) (3) (4) (5) (6) (7) (8) (9) (10)
Energy levels	(1) (2) (3) (4) (5) (6) (7) (8) (9) (10)
Mental clarity	(1) (2) (3) (4) (5) (6) (7) (8) (9) (10)

Feeling sick?

☐ Nope!

☐ Yes...

☐ Nausea   ☐ Diarrhea   ☐ Vomiting   ☐ Sore throat

☐ Congestion   ☐ Coughing   ☐ Chills   ☐ Fever

Other symptoms: _____

LET'S EXPLORE SOME MORE #50

| Hours of Sleep | ① ② ③ ④ ⑤ ⑥ ⑦ ⑧ ⑨ ⑩ ⊕ |
| Sleep Quality | ① ② ③ ④ ⑤ ⑥ ⑦ ⑧ ⑨ ⑩ |

WEATHER

☐ Hot   ☐ Mild   ☐ Cold   BM Pressure: _____

☐ Dry   ☐ Humid   ☐ Wet   Allergen Levels: _____

STRESS LEVELS

| None | Low | Medium | High | Max | @$#%! |

FOOD / MEDICATIONS

FOOD / DRINKS	MEDS / SUPPLEMENTS	TIME	DOSE

☐ usual daily medication

EXERCISE / DAILY ACTIVITY

☐ Damn right, I worked out.

☐ I managed to exercise a bit.

☐ No, I haven't exercised at all.

☐ I did some stuff, and that counts.

DETAILS

NOTES / TRIGGERS / IMPROVEMENTS

_____

_____

_____

WRITE ONE THING YOU'RE GRATEFUL FOR

_____

Date: _____

How are you feeling today?

Like death   Like shit   Not good   Meh   Good   Great!   Amazing!

RATE YOUR PAIN LEVEL

① ② ③ ④ ⑤ ⑥ ⑦ ⑧ ⑨ ⑩

Describe your pain / symptoms

Where do you feel it?

	am	pm
_____	☐	☐
_____	☐	☐
_____	☐	☐
_____	☐	☐
_____	☐	☐
_____	☐	☐
_____	☐	☐
	☐	☐

Front   *Back*

What about your...?

Feeling sick?

Mood	① ② ③ ④ ⑤ ⑥ ⑦ ⑧ ⑨ ⑩
Energy levels	① ② ③ ④ ⑤ ⑥ ⑦ ⑧ ⑨ ⑩
Mental clarity	① ② ③ ④ ⑤ ⑥ ⑦ ⑧ ⑨ ⑩

☐ Nope!

☐ Yes...

☐ Nausea   ☐ Diarrhea   ☐ Vomiting   ☐ Sore throat

☐ Congestion   ☐ Coughing   ☐ Chills   ☐ Fever

Other symptoms: _____

LET'S EXPLORE SOME MORE #51

Hours of Sleep (1)(2)(3)(4)(5)(6)(7)(8)(9)(10)(+)
Sleep Quality (1)(2)(3)(4)(5)(6)(7)(8)(9)(10)

WEATHER

☐ Hot ☐ Mild ☐ Cold BM Pressure: _____

☐ Dry ☐ Humid ☐ Wet Allergen Levels: _____

STRESS LEVELS

None	Low	Medium	High	Max	@$#%!

FOOD / MEDICATIONS

FOOD / DRINKS	MEDS / SUPPLEMENTS	TIME	DOSE
	☐ usual daily medication		

EXERCISE / DAILY ACTIVITY

☐ Damn right, I worked out.

☐ I managed to exercise a bit.

☐ No, I haven't exercised at all.

☐ I did some stuff, and that counts.

DETAILS

NOTES / TRIGGERS / IMPROVEMENTS

_____

_____

_____

WRITE ONE THING YOU'RE GRATEFUL FOR

_____

Date: _____

How are you feeling today?

Like death	Like shit	Not good	Meh	Good	Great!	Amazing!

RATE YOUR PAIN LEVEL

(1) (2) (3) (4) (5) (6) (7) (8) (9) (10)

Describe your pain / symptoms   Where do you feel it?

	am	pm
	☐	☐
	☐	☐
	☐	☐
	☐	☐
	☐	☐
	☐	☐
	☐	☐
	☐	☐

Front   *Back*

What about your...?   Feeling sick?

Mood	① ② ③ ④ ⑤ ⑥ ⑦ ⑧ ⑨ ⑩	☐ Nope!
Energy levels	① ② ③ ④ ⑤ ⑥ ⑦ ⑧ ⑨ ⑩	☐ Yes...
Mental clarity	① ② ③ ④ ⑤ ⑥ ⑦ ⑧ ⑨ ⑩	

☐ Nausea   ☐ Diarrhea   ☐ Vomiting   ☐ Sore throat

☐ Congestion   ☐ Coughing   ☐ Chills   ☐ Fever

Other symptoms: _____

LET'S EXPLORE SOME MORE #52

Hours of Sleep (1) (2) (3) (4) (5) (6) (7) (8) (9) (10) (+)

Sleep Quality (1) (2) (3) (4) (5) (6) (7) (8) (9) (10)

WEATHER

☐ Hot ☐ Mild ☐ Cold BM Pressure: _____

☐ Dry ☐ Humid ☐ Wet Allergen Levels: _____

STRESS LEVELS

None	Low	Medium	High	Max	@$#%!

FOOD / MEDICATIONS

FOOD / DRINKS	MEDS / SUPPLEMENTS	TIME	DOSE
	☐ usual daily medication		

EXERCISE / DAILY ACTIVITY

☐ Damn right, I worked out.

☐ I managed to exercise a bit.

☐ No, I haven't exercised at all.

☐ I did some stuff, and that counts.

DETAILS

NOTES / TRIGGERS / IMPROVEMENTS

WRITE ONE THING YOU'RE GRATEFUL FOR

Date: _____

| Like death | Like shit | Not good | Meh | Good | Great! | Amazing! |

RATE YOUR PAIN LEVEL

① ② ③ ④ ⑤ ⑥ ⑦ ⑧ ⑨ ⑩

Describe your pain / symptoms

Where do you feel it?

	am	pm
_____	☐	☐
_____	☐	☐
_____	☐	☐
_____	☐	☐
_____	☐	☐
_____	☐	☐
_____	☐	☐
_____	☐	☐

Front   *Back*

What about your...?

Feeling sick?

Mood	① ② ③ ④ ⑤ ⑥ ⑦ ⑧ ⑨ ⑩
Energy levels	① ② ③ ④ ⑤ ⑥ ⑦ ⑧ ⑨ ⑩
Mental clarity	① ② ③ ④ ⑤ ⑥ ⑦ ⑧ ⑨ ⑩

☐ Nope!
☐ Yes...

☐ Nausea   ☐ Diarrhea   ☐ Vomiting   ☐ Sore throat
☐ Congestion   ☐ Coughing   ☐ Chills   ☐ Fever

Other symptoms: _____

LET'S EXPLORE SOME MORE #53

Hours of Sleep	① ② ③ ④ ⑤ ⑥ ⑦ ⑧ ⑨ ⑩ ⊕
Sleep Quality	① ② ③ ④ ⑤ ⑥ ⑦ ⑧ ⑨ ⑩

WEATHER

☐ Hot   ☐ Mild   ☐ Cold   BM Pressure: _____

☐ Dry   ☐ Humid   ☐ Wet   Allergen Levels: _____

STRESS LEVELS

None	Low	Medium	High	Max	@$#%!

FOOD / MEDICATIONS

FOOD / DRINKS	MEDS / SUPPLEMENTS	TIME	DOSE
	☐ usual daily medication		

EXERCISE / DAILY ACTIVITY

☐ Damn right, I worked out.

☐ I managed to exercise a bit.

☐ No, I haven't exercised at all.

☐ I did some stuff, and that counts.

DETAILS

NOTES / TRIGGERS / IMPROVEMENTS

_____

_____

_____

WRITE ONE THING YOU'RE GRATEFUL FOR

_____

Date: _____

How are you feeling today?

Like death   Like shit   Not good   Meh   Good   Great!   Amazing!

RATE YOUR PAIN LEVEL
① ② ③ ④ ⑤ ⑥ ⑦ ⑧ ⑨ ⑩

Describe your pain / symptoms

	am	pm
_____	☐	☐
_____	☐	☐
_____	☐	☐
_____	☐	☐
_____	☐	☐
_____	☐	☐
_____	☐	☐
_____	☐	☐

Where do you feel it?

Front   *Back*

What about your...?

Mood	① ② ③ ④ ⑤ ⑥ ⑦ ⑧ ⑨ ⑩
Energy levels	① ② ③ ④ ⑤ ⑥ ⑦ ⑧ ⑨ ⑩
Mental clarity	① ② ③ ④ ⑤ ⑥ ⑦ ⑧ ⑨ ⑩

Feeling sick?

☐ Nope!

☐ Yes...

☐ Nausea   ☐ Diarrhea   ☐ Vomiting   ☐ Sore throat

☐ Congestion   ☐ Coughing   ☐ Chills   ☐ Fever

Other symptoms: _____

LET'S EXPLORE SOME MORE #54

Hours of Sleep ① ② ③ ④ ⑤ ⑥ ⑦ ⑧ ⑨ ⑩ ⊕

Sleep Quality ① ② ③ ④ ⑤ ⑥ ⑦ ⑧ ⑨ ⑩

WEATHER

☐ Hot   ☐ Mild   ☐ Cold   BM Pressure: _____

☐ Dry   ☐ Humid   ☐ Wet   Allergen Levels: _____

STRESS LEVELS

None	Low	Medium	High	Max	@$#%!

FOOD / MEDICATIONS

FOOD / DRINKS	MEDS / SUPPLEMENTS	TIME	DOSE

☐ usual daily medication

EXERCISE / DAILY ACTIVITY

☐ Damn right, I worked out.

☐ I managed to exercise a bit.

☐ No, I haven't exercised at all.

☐ I did some stuff, and that counts.

DETAILS

NOTES / TRIGGERS / IMPROVEMENTS

_____

_____

_____

WRITE ONE THING YOU'RE GRATEFUL FOR

_____

Date: _____

How are you feeling today?

Like death	Like shit	Not good	Meh	Good	Great!	Amazing!

RATE YOUR PAIN LEVEL

① ② ③ ④ ⑤ ⑥ ⑦ ⑧ ⑨ ⑩

Describe your pain / symptoms

Where do you feel it?

	am	pm
_____	☐	☐
_____	☐	☐
_____	☐	☐
_____	☐	☐
_____	☐	☐
_____	☐	☐
_____	☐	☐
_____	☐	☐

Front   *Back*

What about your...?

Mood   ① ② ③ ④ ⑤ ⑥ ⑦ ⑧ ⑨ ⑩
Energy levels   ① ② ③ ④ ⑤ ⑥ ⑦ ⑧ ⑨ ⑩
Mental clarity ① ② ③ ④ ⑤ ⑥ ⑦ ⑧ ⑨ ⑩

Feeling sick?

☐ Nope!
☐ Yes...

☐ Nausea   ☐ Diarrhea   ☐ Vomiting   ☐ Sore throat
☐ Congestion ☐ Coughing   ☐ Chills   ☐ Fever

Other symptoms: _____

LET'S EXPLORE SOME MORE #55

Hours of Sleep ① ② ③ ④ ⑤ ⑥ ⑦ ⑧ ⑨ ⑩ ⊕
Sleep Quality ① ② ③ ④ ⑤ ⑥ ⑦ ⑧ ⑨ ⑩

WEATHER

☐ Hot ☐ Mild ☐ Cold BM Pressure: _____

☐ Dry ☐ Humid ☐ Wet Allergen Levels: _____

STRESS LEVELS

| None | Low | Medium | High | Max | @$#%! |

FOOD / MEDICATIONS

FOOD / DRINKS	MEDS / SUPPLEMENTS	TIME	DOSE
	☐ usual daily medication		

EXERCISE / DAILY ACTIVITY

☐ Damn right, I worked out.

☐ I managed to exercise a bit.

☐ No, I haven't exercised at all.

☐ I did some stuff, and that counts.

DETAILS

NOTES / TRIGGERS / IMPROVEMENTS

WRITE ONE THING YOU'RE GRATEFUL FOR

Date: _____

How are you feeling today?

Like death	Like shit	Not good	Meh	Good	Great!	Amazing!

RATE YOUR PAIN LEVEL

① ② ③ ④ ⑤ ⑥ ⑦ ⑧ ⑨ ⑩

Describe your pain / symptoms

	am	pm
_____	☐	☐
_____	☐	☐
_____	☐	☐
_____	☐	☐
_____	☐	☐
_____	☐	☐
_____	☐	☐
_____	☐	☐

Where do you feel it?

Front   *Back*

What about your...?

Mood	① ② ③ ④ ⑤ ⑥ ⑦ ⑧ ⑨ ⑩
Energy levels	① ② ③ ④ ⑤ ⑥ ⑦ ⑧ ⑨ ⑩
Mental clarity	① ② ③ ④ ⑤ ⑥ ⑦ ⑧ ⑨ ⑩

Feeling sick?

☐ Nope!
☐ Yes...

☐ Nausea ☐ Diarrhea ☐ Vomiting ☐ Sore throat
☐ Congestion ☐ Coughing ☐ Chills ☐ Fever

Other symptoms: _____

LET'S EXPLORE SOME MORE #56

Hours of Sleep　① ② ③ ④ ⑤ ⑥ ⑦ ⑧ ⑨ ⑩ ⊕

Sleep Quality　① ② ③ ④ ⑤ ⑥ ⑦ ⑧ ⑨ ⑩

WEATHER

☐ Hot　　☐ Mild　　☐ Cold　　BM Pressure: _____

☐ Dry　　☐ Humid　☐ Wet　　Allergen Levels: _____

STRESS LEVELS

None	Low	Medium	High	Max	@$#%!

FOOD / MEDICATIONS

FOOD / DRINKS	MEDS / SUPPLEMENTS	TIME	DOSE

☐ usual daily medication

EXERCISE / DAILY ACTIVITY

☐ Damn right, I worked out.

☐ I managed to exercise a bit.

☐ No, I haven't exercised at all.

☐ I did some stuff, and that counts.

DETAILS

NOTES / TRIGGERS / IMPROVEMENTS

WRITE ONE THING YOU'RE GRATEFUL FOR

Date:_____

How are you feeling today?

| Like death | Like shit | Not good | Meh | Good | Great! | Amazing! |

RATE YOUR PAIN LEVEL

① ② ③ ④ ⑤ ⑥ ⑦ ⑧ ⑨ ⑩

Describe your pain / symptoms

Where do you feel it?

	am	pm
	☐	☐
	☐	☐
	☐	☐
	☐	☐
	☐	☐
	☐	☐
	☐	☐
	☐	☐

Front   *Back*

What about your...?

Mood ① ② ③ ④ ⑤ ⑥ ⑦ ⑧ ⑨ ⑩

Energy levels ① ② ③ ④ ⑤ ⑥ ⑦ ⑧ ⑨ ⑩

Mental clarity ① ② ③ ④ ⑤ ⑥ ⑦ ⑧ ⑨ ⑩

Feeling sick?

☐ Nope!

☐ Yes...

☐ Nausea ☐ Diarrhea ☐ Vomiting ☐ Sore throat

☐ Congestion ☐ Coughing ☐ Chills ☐ Fever

Other symptoms:

LET'S EXPLORE SOME MORE #57

Hours of Sleep ① ② ③ ④ ⑤ ⑥ ⑦ ⑧ ⑨ ⑩ ⊕

Sleep Quality ① ② ③ ④ ⑤ ⑥ ⑦ ⑧ ⑨ ⑩

WEATHER

☐ Hot ☐ Mild ☐ Cold BM Pressure: _____

☐ Dry ☐ Humid ☐ Wet Allergen Levels: _____

STRESS LEVELS

None	Low	Medium	High	Max	@$#%!

FOOD / MEDICATIONS

FOOD / DRINKS	MEDS / SUPPLEMENTS	TIME	DOSE

☐ usual daily medication

EXERCISE / DAILY ACTIVITY

☐ Damn right, I worked out.

☐ I managed to exercise a bit.

☐ No, I haven't exercised at all.

☐ I did some stuff, and that counts.

DETAILS

NOTES / TRIGGERS / IMPROVEMENTS

WRITE ONE THING YOU'RE GRATEFUL FOR

Date: _____

How are you feeling today?

Like death	Like shit	Not good	Meh	Good	Great!	Amazing!

RATE YOUR PAIN LEVEL

① ② ③ ④ ⑤ ⑥ ⑦ ⑧ ⑨ ⑩

Describe your pain / symptoms

	am	pm
	☐	☐
	☐	☐
	☐	☐
	☐	☐
	☐	☐
	☐	☐
	☐	☐
	☐	☐

Where do you feel it?

Front *Back*

What about your...?

Mood	① ② ③ ④ ⑤ ⑥ ⑦ ⑧ ⑨ ⑩
Energy levels	① ② ③ ④ ⑤ ⑥ ⑦ ⑧ ⑨ ⑩
Mental clarity	① ② ③ ④ ⑤ ⑥ ⑦ ⑧ ⑨ ⑩

Feeling sick?

☐ Nope!
☐ Yes...

☐ Nausea   ☐ Diarrhea   ☐ Vomiting   ☐ Sore throat
☐ Congestion   ☐ Coughing   ☐ Chills   ☐ Fever

Other symptoms:

LET'S EXPLORE SOME MORE #58

Hours of Sleep   ① ② ③ ④ ⑤ ⑥ ⑦ ⑧ ⑨ ⑩ ⊕

Sleep Quality   ① ② ③ ④ ⑤ ⑥ ⑦ ⑧ ⑨ ⑩

WEATHER

☐   Hot   ☐   Mild   ☐   Cold   BM Pressure: _____

☐   Dry   ☐   Humid   ☐   Wet   Allergen Levels: _____

STRESS LEVELS

None	Low	Medium	High	Max	@$#%!

FOOD / MEDICATIONS

FOOD / DRINKS	MEDS / SUPPLEMENTS	TIME	DOSE
	☐ usual daily medication		

EXERCISE / DAILY ACTIVITY

☐   Damn right, I worked out.

☐   I managed to exercise a bit.

☐   No, I haven't exercised at all.

☐   I did some stuff, and that counts.

DETAILS

NOTES / TRIGGERS / IMPROVEMENTS

_____

_____

_____

WRITE ONE THING YOU'RE GRATEFUL FOR

_____

Date: _____

How are you feeling today?

😝 Like death　😣 Like shit　😠 Not good　🙂 Meh　😀 Good　😁 Great!　😍 Amazing!

RATE YOUR PAIN LEVEL

① ② ③ ④ ⑤ ⑥ ⑦ ⑧ ⑨ ⑩

Describe your pain / symptoms

	am	pm
	☐	☐
	☐	☐
	☐	☐
	☐	☐
	☐	☐
	☐	☐
	☐	☐
	☐	☐

Where do you feel it?

Front　　*Back*

What about your...?

Mood	① ② ③ ④ ⑤ ⑥ ⑦ ⑧ ⑨ ⑩
Energy levels	① ② ③ ④ ⑤ ⑥ ⑦ ⑧ ⑨ ⑩
Mental clarity	① ② ③ ④ ⑤ ⑥ ⑦ ⑧ ⑨ ⑩

Feeling sick?

☐ Nope!
☐ Yes...

☐ Nausea　☐ Diarrhea　☐ Vomiting　☐ Sore throat
☐ Congestion　☐ Coughing　☐ Chills　☐ Fever

Other symptoms:

LET'S EXPLORE SOME MORE #59

Hours of Sleep   ① ② ③ ④ ⑤ ⑥ ⑦ ⑧ ⑨ ⑩ ⊕

Sleep Quality   ① ② ③ ④ ⑤ ⑥ ⑦ ⑧ ⑨ ⑩

WEATHER

☐ Hot   ☐ Mild   ☐ Cold   BM Pressure: _____

☐ Dry   ☐ Humid   ☐ Wet   Allergen Levels: _____

STRESS LEVELS

None	Low	Medium	High	Max	@$#%!

FOOD / MEDICATIONS

FOOD / DRINKS	MEDS / SUPPLEMENTS	TIME	DOSE
	☐ usual daily medication		

EXERCISE / DAILY ACTIVITY

☐ Damn right, I worked out.

☐ I managed to exercise a bit.

☐ No, I haven't exercised at all.

☐ I did some stuff, and that counts.

DETAILS

NOTES / TRIGGERS / IMPROVEMENTS

_____

_____

_____

WRITE ONE THING YOU'RE GRATEFUL FOR

_____

Date:_____

How are you feeling today?

Like death	Like shit	Not good	Meh	Good	Great!	Amazing!

RATE YOUR PAIN LEVEL

① ② ③ ④ ⑤ ⑥ ⑦ ⑧ ⑨ ⑩

Describe your pain / symptoms

	am	pm
	☐	☐
	☐	☐
	☐	☐
	☐	☐
	☐	☐
	☐	☐
	☐	☐
	☐	☐

Where do you feel it?

Front   *Back*

What about your...?

Mood	① ② ③ ④ ⑤ ⑥ ⑦ ⑧ ⑨ ⑩
Energy levels	① ② ③ ④ ⑤ ⑥ ⑦ ⑧ ⑨ ⑩
Mental clarity	① ② ③ ④ ⑤ ⑥ ⑦ ⑧ ⑨ ⑩

Feeling sick?

☐ Nope!

☐ Yes...

☐ Nausea ☐ Diarrhea ☐ Vomiting ☐ Sore throat

☐ Congestion ☐ Coughing ☐ Chills ☐ Fever

Other symptoms:

LET'S EXPLORE SOME MORE #60

Hours of Sleep ① ② ③ ④ ⑤ ⑥ ⑦ ⑧ ⑨ ⑩ ⊕

Sleep Quality ① ② ③ ④ ⑤ ⑥ ⑦ ⑧ ⑨ ⑩

WEATHER

☐ Hot   ☐ Mild   ☐ Cold   BM Pressure: _____

☐ Dry   ☐ Humid   ☐ Wet   Allergen Levels: _____

STRESS LEVELS

None	Low	Medium	High	Max	@$#%!

FOOD / MEDICATIONS

FOOD / DRINKS	MEDS / SUPPLEMENTS	TIME	DOSE

☐ usual daily medication

EXERCISE / DAILY ACTIVITY

☐ Damn right, I worked out.

☐ I managed to exercise a bit.

☐ No, I haven't exercised at all.

☐ I did some stuff, and that counts.

DETAILS

NOTES / TRIGGERS / IMPROVEMENTS

WRITE ONE THING YOU'RE GRATEFUL FOR

Notes

CPSIA information can be obtained
at www.ICGtesting.com
Printed in the USA
LVHW051237010421
683211LV00004B/647